PRACTICAL PRESCRIBING FOR NURSES

PRACTICAL PRESCRIBING FOR NURSES

DEVELOPING COMPETENCY AND SKILL

BARRY STRICKLAND-HODGE
REBECCA DICKINSON
HELEN BRADBURY

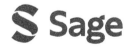 Sage

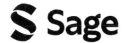

1 Oliver's Yard
55 City Road
London EC1Y 1SP

2455 Teller Road
Thousand Oaks, California 91320

Unit No 323-333, Third Floor, F-Block
International Trade Tower Nehru Place
New Delhi – 110 019

8 Marina View Suite 43-053
Asia Square Tower 1
Singapore 018960

Editor: Laura Walmsley
Editorial Assistant: Sahar Jamfar
Production Editor: Gourav Kumar
Copyeditor: Joy Tucker
Proofreader: Sarah Cooke
Indexer: KnowledgeWorks Global Ltd
Marketing Manager: Ruslana Khatagova
Cover Design: Sheila Tong
Typeset by KnowledgeWorks Global Ltd
Printed and bound by CPI Group (UK) Ltd,
Croydon, CR0 4YY

Library of Congress Control Number: 2023943681

British Library Cataloguing in Publication data

A catalogue record for this book is available from the British Library

ISBN 978-1-5296-0379-8
ISBN 978-1-5296-0378-1 (pbk)

Contents

Abbreviations Used in the Text

ACE	Angiotensin converting enzyme
ADE	Adverse drug event
ADME	Absorption, distribution, metabolism and elimination
ADR	Adverse drug reactions
AKI	Acute kidney injury
AMR	Antimicrobial resistance
APP	Advanced pharmacist practitioner
APPT	Activated partial thromboplastin time
ARR	Absolute risk reduction
BNF	British National Formulary
BNFC	British National Formulary for Children
BSA	Body surface area
CA-MRSA	Community-acquired MRSA
CCG	Clinical commissioning group
CD	Controlled drug
CKD-EPI	Chronic kidney disease epidemiology collaboration
CMO	Chief medical officer
CMP	Clinical management plan
CNS	Central nervous system
COM	Capability and opportunity and motivation
CoP	Community of practice
COX	Cyclooxygenase
CPD	Continuing professional development
CPE	Carbapenemase-producing enterobacterales
CPNP	Community practitioner nurse prescribers
CQC	Care Quality Commission
CQC	Care Quality Commission
CRP	C-reactive protein
DHSS	Department of Health and Social Services (now Department of Health and Social Care)
DOAC	Direct-acting oral anticoagulant
DOH	Department of Health (now Department of Health and Social Care)
eGFR	Estimated glomerular filtration rate

EMC	Electronic Medicines Compendium
EPS	Electronic prescription service
ESBLs	Extended spectrum β-lactamase producing enterobacteriaceae
GFR	Glomerular filtration rate
GI	Gastrointestinal
GMC	General Medical Council
GPhC	General Pharmaceutical Council
HEE	Health Education England
ICBs	Integrated care boards
ICE	Ideas, concerns and expectations
iDAPs	Interactive drug analysis profiles
IgE	Immunoglobulin E
IgG	Immunoglobulin G
INN	International non-proprietary name (used for generic medicines)
INR	International normalised ratio
Lfpse	Learn from patient safety events
LFTs	Liver function tests
LMWH	Low molecular weight heparins
LTC	Long-term conditions
MDT	Multidisciplinary team
MHRA	Medicines and Healthcare products Regulatory Agency
MIC	Minimum inhibitory concentration
MIMS	Monthly Index of Medical Specialities
MAO	Monoamine oxidase
MRI	Magnetic resonance imaging
MRSA	Methicillin-resistant staphylococcus aureus
MST	Morphine sulphate modified release tablets
NEWS2	The latest version of National Early Warning Score
NHS	National Health Service
NICE	National Institute for Health and Care Excellence
NMC	Nursing and Midwifery Council
NNT	Numbers needed to treat
NPC	National Prescribing Centre
NPF	Nurse Prescribers' Formulary
NPSA	National Patient Safety Agency
NQN	Newly qualified nurse
NRLS	National Reporting and Learning System
NSAIDs	Non-steroidal anti-inflammatory drugs
PACT	Prescribing analysis and cost
PCN	Primary care networks
PCT	Procalcitonin
PGD	Patient group direction
PIL	Patient information leaflet
PIM	Potentially inappropriate medicine
POC	Point of care

POM	Prescription-only medicine
PPE	Personal protective equipment
PPIs	Proton pump inhibitors
PSD	Patient-specific direction
QOF	Quality and outcomes frameworks
RCN	Royal College of Nursing
RPS	Royal Pharmaceutical Society
SE	Side-effect
SmPC	Summary of Product Characteristics
SPS	Specialist Pharmacy Service
UKCPA	United Kingdom Clinical Pharmacy Association
UKHSA	United Kingdom Health Security Agency
UTI	Urinary tract infection
v/v	Volume in or per volume
V100	Prescribing programme as part of a specialist practitioner qualification.
V200	Extended formulary nurse prescribers
V300	Nurse independent/supplementary prescribers
w/v	Weight in (or per) volume
w/w	Weight in or per weight
WCC	White cell count
WHO	World Health Organization

About the Editors

Barry Strickland-Hodge MSc, PhD, FRPharmS, FHEA, Visiting Professor of Prescribing Practice at the University of Leeds and a doctoral supervisor for students at the university of Derby. He was a prescribing adviser to GP practices in Newham and Belfast for 15 years. He developed the prescribing course for pharmacists at the University of Leeds in 2003, with the first intake in 2004. Barry has an interest in the history of medicine and pharmacy and became an apothecary in 1990. He has written a number of books and papers on prescribing and information systems.

Rebecca Dickinson PhD, RGN, is programme lead for adult nursing at the University of Leeds and Chair of the School Ethics Committee. She supports teaching on the independent and supplementary prescribing course for nurses and midwives. Rebecca is interested in how to optimally support patients with understanding about taking their medicines and has a particular interest in promoting understanding of how risk of harm, likelihood of benefit and uncertainty about medicines are communicated to patients. Rebecca's PhD was jointly supported by the University of Leeds and the MHRA and focused on the provision of a headline section and additional benefit information in regulated patient information leaflets.

Helen Bradbury BSc., (Pharm)., MEd., FRPharmS., FHEA., Visiting Associate Professor at the University of Leeds. Helen worked in the NHS as a hospital pharmacist for 20 years before commencing her academic career. Helen's subject specialities are clinical education, with an interest in pharmacy education, personal and professional development and interprofessional education. In her last role as professional lead for pharmacy she advised on the delivery of the independent prescribing programmes for nurses, midwives, pharmacists and allied healthcare professionals. She has published on reflective practice, interprofessional education and prescribing for medical students.

About the Contributors

Sue Alldred MAPCPharm, MRPharmS, BPharm(Hons), PGDipClinPharm, Independent Prescriber, Advanced Pharmacist Practitioner working in a medical centre and Head of Clinical Pharmacy for South and East Leeds GP group. She is a practising prescriber working across the breadth of clinical conditions encountered in primary care. Prior to this she was a specialist neurology pharmacist at Leeds Teaching Hospitals. She is the regional vice-president for the Primary Care Pharmacists Association and teaches and mentors both postgraduate pharmacists and trainees and pharmacy technicians, together with working as a designated prescribing practitioner for trainee prescribers.

Natalie Bryars BPharm, PGDipClinPharm, Med, MRPharmS, Principal Pharmacist in Clinical Governance at York and Scarborough Teaching Hospitals NHS Foundation Trust. Natalie's role spans clinical governance in secondary care and quality assurance of pharmacy services. She focuses on medicines management, where she writes and reviews policies and procedures, assesses and audits compliance with standards, produces and delivers training programmes and assures the delivery of quality services. She has a keen interest in prescribing and contributes to the prescribing programme for the Hull and York Medical School; her research has focused on how prescribing can be taught more effectively to medical students. She also contributes to the governance and education programmes for non-medical prescribers within her organisation.

Claire Easthall PhD, MPharm, MRPharmS, FHEA, is a Lecturer in Pharmacy in the School of Healthcare, University of Leeds. She is Programme Lead for the PGDip in Pharmacy and also supports teaching and assessment on the Independent Prescribing course. Claire is interested in health behaviour change, with a specific focus on supporting optimal medicines use via person-centred approaches to care and understanding medicines use as a complex health behaviour. Her PhD focused on development of a screening tool to identify individual patient barriers to medicines adherence, yielding a range of peer-reviewed publications. Claire's teaching expertise is integrated into her research interests, but also covers areas such as consultation skills, professional development and reflective practice.

Daniel Greer BPharm, MSc (Clin Pharm), PGCert (Clinical Education), Lead Pharmacist for Gastroenterology, Leeds Teaching Hospitals NHS Trust and formerly Teacher Practitioner on the postgraduate programme in Pharmacy Practice in the School of Healthcare, University of Leeds. He also contributed to teaching pharmacology within the school.

Lorraine Henshaw DPrac (nursing), MSc, RN, RNT, SFHEA, is a registered general nurse with experience in a variety of clinical and educational settings including neonatal intensive care, general practice nursing and as a clinical research nurse. Currently her role is as a Senior Lecturer in Nursing and Advanced Clinical Practice at the University of Staffordshire. Her research interests centre upon workforce development, role transition and nurse identity.

Joseph Spencer-Jones MRPharmS, PGDip, PGCert, Advanced Clinical Pharmacist for Antimicrobials at Mid Yorkshire Teaching Trust. A qualified pharmacist for ten years, he took a keen interest in antimicrobials when working in infectious diseases at Leeds Teaching Hospitals. An Independent Prescriber from the University of Leeds, he now delivers teaching on the Antimicrobials syllabus for this course. Joe is currently building his research portfolio, with a keen interest in optimising the use of antimicrobials.

Melanie McGinlay BSc (Hons), MSc, Lecturer and Visiting Researcher at the University of Leeds, Leeds Institute of Cardiovascular and Metabolic Medicine and heart failure specialist nurse at Leeds Teaching Hospitals. Melanie has been a registered nurse in cardiology for 14 years and led on the independent and supplementary prescribing course for pharmacists, allied health professionals, midwives and nurses at the University of Leeds. She has written and co-authored on a number of peer-reviewed research papers with a particular focus on medicines optimisation of disease-modifying therapy in chronic cardiac conditions.

Daniel Okeowo MPharm, MRPharmS, is a Lecturer of Pharmacy Practice at Newcastle University and a PhD candidate at the University of Leeds. His research focuses on 'How can deprescribing be safely routinely implemented in primary care?' With a background as a practising pharmacist in primary care, Daniel brings valuable expertise to his research. His research interests lie in polypharmacy and exploring the practical implementation of deprescribing strategies. Furthermore, Daniel has experience teaching various disciplines, including pharmacy, nursing, medicine and postgraduate prescriber courses.

Ruth Setchell (Margaret) BSc (Pharm), PG Cert in Psychiatric Therapeutics. Recently retired from a 35-year career as a hospital pharmacist. After specialising in aseptic services, Ruth changed direction and moved into psychiatric pharmacy, adding a certificate in psychiatric therapeutics from Aston University to her clinical pharmacy diploma. From managing a small psychiatric pharmacy team Ruth subsequently joined a multidisciplinary care homes team project to reduce antipsychotic prescribing in residents with dementia. She qualified as an Independent Prescriber and prescribed psychotropic medications for patients of the care homes team. Throughout her career she has been involved in training clinical, medical, nursing and allied professionals, teaching pre-registration pharmacists, clinical pharmacists and technicians on various programmes within hospitals, universities and with CPPE. She co-authored 'Managing Behavioural and Psychological Disturbance in Dementia', a guidance and resource pack for Leeds in 2014.

Acknowledgements

Agnes Kozlowska. MHRA Customer Experience Centre, Communications and Engagement

Alexandra Freeman. NHSE/Winton Centre for Risk & Evidence Communication, University of Cambridge

Angela Crawford. Directorate Administrator Royal Pharmaceutical Society

Datapharm Professional Regulation Directorate

Emma Blankson. Policy Manager, General Medical Council

House of Commons Library

Ian Moir. National Institute for Health and Care Excellence, Science, Evidence and Analytics Directorate

Jane Trodd. Royal Pharmaceutical Society Librarian

Medicines and Healthcare Products Regulatory Agency

Nursing and Midwifery Council Education and Standards Team

Penny North-Lewis. Leeds Teaching Hospitals NHS Trust

Rebecca Braybrooks. Royal Pharmaceutical Society Professional Support Adviser

Specialist Pharmacy Services

The Leeds Library

Introduction

As I write this, it is 350 years since Jonathan Goddard, a London physician, wrote 'only doctors should prescribe' (Goddard, 1670). This was at a time when he and many other physicians were railing against the apothecaries who had increased their level of involvement in the prescribing of medicines. When there were few physicians in London, such as in times of sickness, illness and plague, the apothecaries felt it necessary to take on the role not only of compounding and dispensing, but also diagnosing and prescribing. In 1968, still 300 years after Goddard, the Medicines Act of 1968 stated that under the National Health Service the only individuals who would be able to prescribe would be doctors and dentists for patients and veterinary surgeons for animals. Even so, dentists were required to use the *Dental Practitioners' Formulary* if they were to prescribe for their NHS patients. Privately dentists were allowed to prescribe anything they felt was appropriate and for which they felt they had the knowledge.

It wasn't until 1986 that Baroness Cumberlege, in the House of Lords, moved that community nurses, including district nurses, should be allowed to prescribe from a specific shortlist of medicines for their patients. This was supported in the Lords and in the Commons because it was realised that district nurses, for example, requiring dressing packs or similar would need to get a prescription signed by a doctor. After this – which might seem a small change, but did require new legislation – things moved much more rapidly as Dr June Crown produced the Crown reports recommending that others should be able to prescribe. In April 2012 a major change took place: that qualified independent prescribing nurses and independent prescribing pharmacists were permitted to prescribe anything from the *British National Formulary* (BNF) within their scope of practice, with two specific exemptions when used for addiction. It was only a matter of time before other healthcare professionals, following a regulated prescribing course, were permitted to prescribe from a range of medicines for their patients, with certain specific restrictions.

This short book looks at various aspects of prescribing, from its history to the transition from qualified nurse to prescriber. It includes deprescribing, where medicines considered inappropriate can be, with the patient's involvement and agreement, removed from a list of repeat prescriptions.

One important aspect of this book is that we do not define prescribing by what it is not. You will not see the letters *non*, related to prescribing or the prescribers you are, or will become. We are all expected to follow the *Competency Framework for All Prescribers* published by the Royal Pharmaceutical Society in 2021. These show the skills and competencies that all prescribers from whatever branch of healthcare they come should be able to demonstrate.

In fact, this book follows the competency framework closely. Each chapter takes aspects of the framework and explains and describes what these mean in practice. Each chapter, following the history of nurse prescribing, is broken down into various parts, but all in some way relate to the framework.

We hope you will find this book useful before, during and after courses in prescribing.

Barry Strickland-Hodge
Pharmacist, apothecary and visiting professor of prescribing practice

References

Goddard, J.A. 1670. *Discourse, setting forth the unhappy condition of the practice of physick in London*. London: Royal Society, VIII, 442–55. The London Physician found at the Leeds Subscription Library.

1

The Development of
Nurse Prescribing

Barry Strickland-Hodge

Chapter summary

This chapter presents the history of nurse involvement in prescribing. It starts with the Cumberlege report of 1986, which recommended nurse prescribing, and includes two essential Crown reports of the early 1990s further supporting this recommendation. From there, it looks at the inclusion of professional groups other than nurses before the eventual prescribing availability of all medicines within the *British National Formulary* (BNF) (with a few specific exceptions) by nurses from 2012.

The chapter will also introduce the development of different ways of making medicines more easily available to patients including administration, supply and prescribing including:

- patient-specific directions (PSD)
- patient group directions (PGDs)
- clinical management plans (CMP)
- supplementary prescribing
- independent prescribing.

Finally, the chapter will explore the Nursing and Midwifery Council (NMC) *Standards of Proficiency for Registered Nurses* and the development of the curriculum to include aspects of prescribing for nurse education. For context, it will also include a brief discussion of prescribing for pharmacists and allied health professionals who you will be working with.

Introduction

There are some nurses, particularly those who have recently entered the profession, who might think prescribing has always been part of nurses' activity. Those nurses who have been in the profession longer will know this is not the case.

The Medicines Act of 1968 first defined prescribers as doctors and dentists (and veterinary surgeons for animals). However, long before the Medicines Act, in fact in 1670, one physician had already said only doctors should prescribe (Goddard, 1670).

In this chapter we will look back over the introduction of a limited level of prescribing for community nurses and conclude with the independent nurse prescriber having rights to prescribe, with very limited exceptions, all medicines within the *British National Formulary* (BNF) – always acting professionally and within their scope of practice and knowledge.

The start of nurse prescribing: The Cumberlege report

The Cumberlege report of 1986 discusses all aspects of nursing in the community making recommendations on each aspect.

In the Foreword, it references a 1985 survey which found that: 'Nurses (working in the community) were at their most effective when they and general practitioners worked together in an active primary healthcare team' (Cumberlege, 1986, Foreword). This was a new concept in 1986; it goes on to say, 'We would like to see the introduction into primary healthcare of the nurse practitioner' (Cumberlege, 1986, Foreword). And again, very briefly, it says, 'We also recommend that community nurses should be able to prescribe a limited range of items and simple agents and to control drug dosage in certain well-defined circumstances' (Cumberlege, 1986, Foreword).

Baroness Cumberlege realised that this may require some legislation but in general she tried to avoid anything that would involve changes in the law. This is the first time that the concept of nurses in the community being able to prescribe was mentioned in an official government-sponsored report.

In the summary of recommendations, recommendation 7 states: 'The DHSS should agree a limited list of items and simple agents which may be prescribed by nurses as part of a nursing care programme and issue guidelines to enable nurses to control drug dosage in well-defined circumstances' (Cumberlege, 1986, p. 62). Most of what we now have, developed from this simple recommendation.

The whole ethos of what Baroness Cumberlege was trying to achieve was to:

> Provide support in the community so that as far as possible, hospital admission is prevented, early discharge from hospital is encouraged, people with permanent health problems could remain in their own homes and people who are terminally ill could, if they wished, be allowed to die at home.
>
> (Cumberlege, 1986, p. 8)

Under a section of the report entitled 'New roles', nurse practitioners are described as a fundamental part of the whole system. However, they were not seen as such before this report was written. It is possible that nurse practitioners may have existed in specific districts but not as an identified profession. Baroness Cumberlege states:

> Research has shown that nurses could be as effective as doctors and as acceptable to patients in securing compliance with therapy for chronic disease, making initial assessments of patients, diagnosing and treating certain minor acute illnesses and behavioural disorders and rehabilitating elderly people after surgery. (Cumberlege, 1986, p. 31)

Cumberlege was concentrating on simple basic skills whereas now we look at nurse practitioners or nurse prescribers as much more skilled and as full members of the community care team.

A key point and the initial consideration that led to nurse prescribing was probably outlined halfway through the report. There is a very short section, two paragraphs plus a recommendation, called 'Power to prescribe'. Quoting from the report it says, 'We found district nurses waste time in requesting prescriptions from general practitioners for such things as dressings, ointments and medical sprays for those with leg ulcers for example' (Cumberlege, 1986, p. 33). She goes on to say that in addition, many nurses have become very skilled in managing pain relief for terminally ill patients. The report states: 'We believe therefore that community nurses who work with terminally ill patients should be permitted to use their professional judgement on matters such as the timing and dosage of drugs prescribed for pain relief' (Cumberlege, 1986, p. 33).

Think about nurse prescribing now, where an independent fully trained nurse prescriber has access to the whole of the BNF, working within their scope of practice. It is important to realise that this was groundbreaking.

The Crown reports

In 1989, a report of the Advisory Group on Nurse Prescribing chaired by Dr June Crown (Department of Health) endorsed nurse prescribing and highlighted the circumstances in which it could occur. A successful private member's bill proposed by Sir (then Mr) Roger Sims in the House of Commons and moved by Baroness Cumberlege in the House of Lords led to the primary legislation Medicinal Products: Prescription By Nurses Etc. Act 1992, which provided the legal framework for nurses to prescribe.

The list of products that were permitted under the *Nurse Prescribers' Formulary* (NPF) to be prescribed by community nurses who had undergone the necessary training is relatively brief, but it enabled the nurse to prescribe in areas such as minor injuries, minor ailments, health promotion and palliative care.

In 1998 Dr June Crown again chaired a review considering the supply and administration of medicines under what were called group protocols. These protocols were defined as: 'General guidelines written or agreed by doctors under which specified medicines are administered or supplied by other health professionals to patients in defined clinical circumstances' (Crown, 1998, Appendix D, p. 12). The review discovered a wide variety of group protocols being used across the country and what they were expected to cover and permit.

The problem was that although they had evolved for very good reasons, including reducing patient waiting times, they were varied across the country and the legality of these arrangements had been called into question by the Department of Health. The review therefore wanted to maintain the overall ethos of the protocols but made strong recommendations to create legal, standard protocols which are now known as patient group directions (PGDs).

Processes for the administration, supply and prescribing of medicines

Administration: The **patient-specific direction (PSD)**

A prescription for a named patient is a particular patient-specific direction informing the pharmacist what needs to be dispensed and for whom. The broader term 'patient-specific direction' can be for more than one patient being seen by a nurse or other healthcare professional. It is an instruction to administer a medicine to a list of individually named patients. The list has the names of each patient who will be seen and the name of the person who will be administering the medicine. It is signed by the registered prescriber who should have adequate knowledge of the patients on the list.

The PSD can be for any medicine including vaccinations to be administered after the prescriber has assessed the patient on an individual basis. This assessment can be via the patient's record.

A verbal instruction is not a valid PSD. As the responsibility for any PSD rests with the prescriber, the prescriber will clearly need to be satisfied that the person to whom they give the instruction is competent to administer the medicine concerned.

The patient-specific direction is often used in clinics where a number of named patients are coming to have a procedure – for example, to see an ophthalmologist. The named nurse or other professional on the PSD is permitted by the signature of the prescriber in charge of the clinic to administer, for example, eye drops prior to the patient going in to see the ophthalmologist.

Supply: Patient group direction (PGD)

Whereas a prescription and PSD are for named patients, a patient group direction is for a named drug or medicine. It is a concise document giving the name of medicine, the patient groups it can be supplied to (and those for whom it is contraindicated), the name of the nurse or other healthcare professional and enough information on which to base a decision to supply the medicine such as which age groups it can be used for, for how long and what information the supplier needs to record, such as batch numbers and expiry dates of the medicine. Each PGD is signed by a senior doctor and pharmacist and any other specific prescriber who may be recommended, such as the community paediatrician for children's medicines.

They have been used extensively and have shown their usefulness particularly in places like walk-in centres. Following a patient consultation and examination, medicines can be supplied under the strict rules of the PGD. The person supplying must only do this within the scope of their practice. PGDs are written by a senior pharmacist in conjunction with a senior medic within the geographic area, such as a clinical commissioning group.

Question 1.1

What are the differences between a PSD and a PGD? See **Answer 1.1**

Answer 1.1

The obvious difference is that PSDs are patient-specific, even if there is more than one patient on the list. PSDs, on the one hand, are designed for administration of medicine, not supply. They are signed by the prescriber in charge of the clinic who takes responsibility overall.

PGDs, on the other hand, are legal documents developed from group protocols. They are medicine-specific and are so that the person named on the PGD can supply. They are signed by a senior doctor and pharmacist and the name of the person working within the PGD must be on the document.

PSDs are often used in clinics where named patients are to be seen. PGDs are used in many places, including walk-in centres, for supply of medicine.

Prescribing is different

The final Crown report of 1999 recommended that other defined health professionals, following specific training, should be able to prescribe for patients. There would be two types of prescribers: *independent* and *dependent*. The latter term was later changed to *supplementary* prescriber.

Supplementary prescribing (formerly dependent prescribing)

The Crown report defined this as: 'a voluntary partnership between an independent prescriber (a doctor or dentist) and a supplementary prescriber to implement an agreed patient-specific Clinical Management Plan (CMP) with the patient's agreement' (BNF, 2023).The CMP is integral to this form of prescribing. See **Box 1.1** for full details of what a CMP needs to contain.

Supplementary prescribers can prescribe anything within their scope of practice that has been initially approved and written onto a clinical management plan (CMP). In this case the independent prescriber remains the doctor or dentist. There are a number of conditions for the nurse to act as a supplementary prescriber. There is a course to be undertaken and the CMP itself has to contain specific information. What a CMP must contain is shown in **Box 1.1**. The independent and supplementary prescriber must agree to the use of the CMP for named patients as this is a voluntary relationship, but the patient must also agree to be treated by the supplementary prescriber in this way.

Box 1.1

A clinical management plan must contain the following information:

a. the name of the patient to whom the plan relates;
b. the illnesses or conditions which may be treated by the supplementary prescriber;

---

c. the date on which the plan is to take effect and when it is to be reviewed by the doctor or dentist who is a party to the plan;

d. reference to the class or description of medicinal product which may be prescribed or administered under the plan;

e. any restrictions or limitations as to the strength or dose of any product which may be prescribed or administered under the plan, and any period of administration or use of any medicinal product which may be prescribed or administered under the plan;

f. relevant warnings about the known sensitivities of the patient to, or known difficulties of the patient with, particular medicinal products;

g. the arrangements for notification of:
   - suspected or known adverse reactions to any medicinal product which may be prescribed or administered under the plan; and
   - suspected or known adverse reactions to any other medicinal product taken at the same time as any medicinal product prescribed or administered under the plan;

h. the circumstances in which the supplementary prescriber should refer to, or seek the advice of, the doctor or dentist who is a party to the plan.

Independent prescribing

This is prescribing by an appropriate practitioner (e.g., doctor, dentist, nurse, pharmacist; see **Box 1.2** for full list) responsible and accountable for the assessment of patients with undiagnosed or diagnosed conditions and for decisions about the clinical management required, including prescribing.

Prescribing for community practitioners and nurse prescribers

In summary, community practitioners, who have not qualified as supplementary or independent prescribers, can prescribe from the NPF in the BNF (see Chapter 2). They cannot prescribe controlled drugs (CDs) or unlicensed drugs, which we will discuss in Chapter 10. Supplementary prescribers work within a CMP and, from April 2012, qualified independent nurse prescribers could prescribe from the whole BNF, with one or two minor exclusions for addiction (see **Box 1.2** for a full list of potential prescribers and any restrictions on their prescribing).

So you can see that to get to this position took a number of motivated and dedicated individuals such as Baroness Cumberlege, Sir Roger Sims, Dr June Crown and a willing Department of Health to enable nurse prescribing. From the NPF came the next stage where prescribing was broadened and further defined, and the range of nurses enabled to prescribe was also increased from community nurse practitioners to all fully trained nurses.

The final stage was permitting the fully qualified nurse, following a specific NMC-approved prescribing course at a university including practical experience, to prescribe from the whole of the BNF (with one or two exceptions) working within their own scope of practice. The list of those who can now be trained and prescribe and any restrictions on what they can prescribe are shown in **Box 1.2**.

Box 1.2 Who can prescribe?

Prescribers other than doctors, dentists and, for animals other than humans, veterinary surgeons are currently:

- nurse and midwife independent prescribers, but cocaine, diamorphine or dipipanone is not permitted if used for treating addiction;
- optometrist independent prescribers (though they cannot prescribe CDs or unlicensed medicines and the prescriptions must be for treating conditions affecting the eye and surrounding tissue only);
- paramedics but they cannot yet prescribe CDs or unlicensed preparations;
- pharmacists but cocaine, diamorphine or dipipanone is not permitted if used for treating addiction;
- physiotherapists with restrictions on the specific CDs, no unlicensed medicines;
- podiatrists who again have specific CDs they can prescribe and no unlicensed medicines;
- therapeutic radiographers but no CDs or unlicensed preparations.

Remember, this list stemmed from an initial consideration for a very limited list of preparations for community practitioners only.

As discussed above, the primary legislation that enables nurses and midwives to prescribe is the Medicinal Products: Prescription By Nurses Etc. Act 1992. In this Act, nurses, midwives and health visitors were enabled to prescribe for the first time.

The Nursing and Midwifery Council (NMC) published the *Standards of Proficiency for Nurse and Midwife Prescribers*, which was updated when the new Royal Pharmaceutical Society framework was published in 2021. However, there were some important points in 2006, particularly around definitions of specific nursing groups, which are important (see **Box 1.3**).

Box 1.3

Previous definition	Current definition
District nurse/health visitor formulary nurses and any nurse undertaking a V100 prescribing programme as part of a specialist practitioner qualification	Community practitioner nurse prescribers (V100)
Extended formulary nurse prescribers	Nurse independent prescribers (V200 only)
Extended/supplementary nurse prescribers	Nurse independent/supplementary prescribers (V300)

The NMC Code, Professional Standards of Practice and Behaviour for Nurses, Midwives and Nursing Associates, was published in 2015 and updated in 2018 (see **Box 1.4** for details).

Box 1.4

Section 18 of the Code states: 'Advise on, prescribe, supply, dispense or administer medicines within the limits of your training and competence, the law, our guidance and other relevant policies, guidance and regulations.'

To achieve this, you must:

- prescribe, advise on, or provide medicines or treatment, including repeat prescriptions (only if you are suitably qualified) if you have enough knowledge of that person's health and are satisfied that the medicines or treatment serve that person's health needs;
- keep to appropriate guidelines when giving advice on using controlled drugs and recording the prescribing, supply, dispensing or administration of controlled drugs;
- make sure that the care or treatment you advise on, prescribe, supply, dispense or administer for each person is compatible with any other care or treatment they are receiving, including (where possible) over-the-counter medicines;
- take all steps to keep medicines stored securely;
- wherever possible, avoid prescribing for yourself or for anyone with whom you have a close personal relationship.

Prescribing is not within the scope of practice of everyone on our register. Nursing associates don't prescribe, but they may supply, dispense and administer medicines. Nurses and midwives who have successfully completed a further qualification in prescribing and recorded it on our register are the only people on our register that can prescribe (NMC, 2015, updated 2018).

The current position

Some of you may have heard the term 'prescribing ready' and wondered if that meant you would be able to prescribe when you graduated and registered. This is not the case. As the NMC stated 'the law clearly states that nurses can only undertake a prescribing qualification post-registration'. See **Box 1.5** for the relevant section of *Future Nurse* proficiencies.

Box 1.5

However, the key standards in the *Future Nurse* proficiencies stated that *at the point of qualification and registration* a newly qualified nurse (NQN) would be able to do the following:

- understand the principles of safe and effective administration and optimisation of medicines in accordance with local and national policies and demonstrate proficiency and accuracy when calculating dosages of prescribed medicines;

- demonstrate knowledge of pharmacology and the ability to recognise the effects of medicines, allergies, drug sensitivities, side-effects, contraindications, incompatibilities, adverse reactions, prescribing errors and the impact of polypharmacy and over-the-counter medication usage;
- demonstrate knowledge of how prescriptions can be generated, the role of generic, unlicensed and off-label prescribing (see Chapter 10) and an understanding of the potential risks associated with these approaches to prescribing;
- apply knowledge of pharmacology to the care of people, demonstrating the ability to progress to a prescribing qualification following registration.

So, although not able to prescribe, the NQN would be able to apply to attend a recognised prescribing course earlier than was originally agreed. With the introduction of these updated, more advanced proficiencies for registered nurses, the NMC considered that it would no longer be necessary to insist on such lengthy periods on the register (three years) before allowing nurses to progress to undertake prescribing programmes as had been the case previously.

Under the 2018 Standards for Prescribing Programmes, therefore, it was agreed that it would be permissible for nurses to undertake a recognised short course to progress to V100/V150 community prescribing qualifications immediately after registration, and to a V300 independent prescribing qualification after having been registered with the NMC for a minimum period of one year, providing all other entry requirements are met in full.

Following a survey of its members, the Royal College of Nursing had a caveat:

> We agreed in principle that there could be a reduction in the current 3-year requirement before registrants could complete the supplementary/independent prescriber (known as V300), but the individual practitioner and the context in which they work will need to be considered. Not all settings require nurses to have V300. It is essential that a formal programme of health assessment has been obtained beforehand; so realistically, we felt it would be difficult to complete the training in less than two years. (RCN, 2017)

Many courses approved at the time of writing still have the three-year requirement following registration before the registered nurse or midwife could undertake the prescribing course, although as nursing students are beginning to qualify under the *Future Nurse* standards some courses have begun to amend this requirement to one-year post-qualification experience in a patient-focused role. It is expected that this will be reduced for those nurses and midwives nationally already qualified once the transition to the new undergraduate NMC-approved courses has been achieved.

Summary

We have come a long way from the Cumberlege report of 1986 and the Crown reviews, reports and recommendations. Nurses paved the way for other healthcare professionals to prescribe and supply medicines. University courses are NMC-approved and offer places to appropriate nurses to undertake the prescribing course with the view of prescribing as an independent nurse or midwife prescriber. It is a great hard-won responsibility, and you must always work within your scope of practice and seek further information if necessary through continuing professional development, which is discussed a little later in this book.

References

BNF 2023. *Non-medical Prescribing*. Available at bnf.nice.org.uk/guidance/non-medical-prescribing/html (accessed 12 May 2023).

Crown, J. 1998. *Review of Prescribing, Supply and Administration of Medicines: A Report on the Supply and Administration of Medicines under Groups Protocols*. London: Department of Health.

Crown, J. 1999. *Review of Prescribing, Supply and Administration of Medicines: Final Report*. London: Department of Health.

Cumberlege, J. 1986. *Neighbourhood Nursing: A Focus for Care. Report of the Community Nursing Review*. London: Department of Health, HMSO.

Cumberlege, J. 1992. Second reading. Medicinal Products: Prescription By Nurses Etc Bill. Volume 536: debated on Friday 28 February.

Department of Health (DoH) 1989. *Report of the Advisory Group on Nurse Prescribing*. London: Department of Health. (Chaired by Dr June Crown).

Goddard, J.A. 1670. *Discourse, setting forth the unhappy condition of the practice of physick in London*. London: Royal Society, VIII, 442–55.

Human Medicines Regulation Act 2012. London: HMSO.

Medicinal Products: Prescription By Nurses Etc. Act 1992 (C. 28). [online] London: HMSO. Available at www.legislation.gov.uk/ukpga/1992/28 (accessed 12 May 2023).

Medicines Act 1968 (C. 67). [online] London: HMSO. Available at www.legislation.gov.uk/ukpga/1968/67/contents (accessed 12 May 2023).

NMC 2015, updated 2018. *Code of Professional Standards of Practice and Behaviour for Nurses, Midwives and Nursing Associates*. London: NMC.

NMC 2018. *Future Nurse: Standards of Proficiency for Registered Nurses*. London: NMC. Available at www.nmc.org.uk/globalassets/sitedocuments/standards-of-proficiency/nurses/future-nurse-proficiencies.pdf (accessed 12 May 2023).

NPF 2022. *Nurse Prescribers' Formulary*. Available at bnf.nice.org.uk/nurse-prescribers-formulary/ (accessed 21 May 2023).

RCN 2017. *The Royal College of Nursing (RCN's) response to the NMC consultations on: Standards of proficiency for registered nurses*. Available at www.rcn.org.uk/-/media/Royal-College-Of-Nursing/Documents/Publications/2017/Ocotber/PDF-006505.pdf (accessed 12 May 2023).

A Competency Framework for all Prescribers Royal Pharmaceutical Society (2021).

Sims, R. 1992. Private member's bill. HC Deb. vol. 202 cols. 1196–234, 31 January 1992. Available at www.theyworkforyou.com/debates/?id=1992-01-31a.1196.0 (accessed 12 May 2023).

2

Prescribing Resources and Competency Frameworks

Barry Strickland-Hodge

Chapter summary

This chapter discusses:

- formularies
- the *British National Formulary* (BNF) and the *British National Formulary for Children* (BNFC)
- the Drug Tariff
- *Electronic Medicines Compendium* (EMC)
- the *Nurse Prescribers' Formulary* (NPF) for V100 and V150 prescribers
- competency frameworks generally and
- the *Competency Framework for All Prescribers*.

Introduction

As you have seen from Chapter 1, prescribing – from 1968 following the publication of the Medicines Act (Medicines Act, 1968) until the publication of the Medicinal Products: Prescription By Nurses Etc. Act (1992) – was the realm of doctors and dentists only (and vets for animals). Following the publication of this latter Act in 1992 (Medicinal Products, 1992) community practitioner nurse prescribers could prescribe from a limited list of medicinal products: the *Nurse Prescribers' Formulary for Community Practitioners* (NPF). There have been many formularies particularly in hospital but the ones we will start with are the NPF and the *British National Formulary* (BNF). Formal frameworks for prescribers have been available since 2001; the first for nurse prescribers will be discussed, ending with the latest RPS publication *A Competency Framework for All Prescribers* (RPS, 2021). The competencies being discussed in this chapter are: Competency 4, Prescribe, with the statement supporting the competency being, '4.3. Understands and uses relevant national, regional and local frameworks for the use of medicines'; and Competency 8, Prescribe Professionally, with the supporting statement, '8.3. Knows and works within legal and regulatory frameworks affecting prescribing practice'.

In the Further information section of the *Competency Framework* (in the supporting statements for Competency 4 and Competency 8) it says, 'frameworks include local formularies, care pathways, protocols and professional guidelines, as well as evidence-based guidelines from relevant national, regional and local committees' (RPS, 2021). Thus the inclusion of frameworks and formularies here.

Formularies

In the UK, formularies exist to specify which drugs are available on the NHS for particular groups of prescribers. The two main reference sources providing this information are the BNF and the Drug Tariff; both are available online as an app or in hard copy (see also Chapter 1). In hospital, formularies are a method by which physicians and pharmacists, working through an appropriate medicines committee, can evaluate and select medications for use in the hospital.

Local NHS hospital trusts and integrated care boards (ICBs) often produce their own list of medicines considered best for prescribing within their organisation or the whole locality. It would be particularly useful if such formularies created through medicines committees in hospital were shared with primary care to help when transferring patients from hospital. This is done in some areas but not all.

Local formularies across England vary in the range of medicines the formulary includes and the processes for developing and updating the formulary. A list of potential benefits of local formularies is shown in **Box 2.1**.

The *British National Formulary* (BNF)

You will have come across the BNF on many occasions, and it was mentioned in Chapter 1 of this book. It contains a wide spectrum of information and advice on prescribing and

> ## Box 2.1
>
> Benefits of local formularies may include:
>
> - improving patient outcomes by optimising the use of medicines;
> - supporting the inclusion of patient factors in decisions about medicines;
> - improving local care pathways;
> - improving collaboration between health professionals and commissioners;
> - improving quality by reducing inappropriate variations in clinical care;
> - improving quality through access to cost-effective medicines;
> - supporting the supply of medicines across a local health economy;
> - supporting financial management and expenditure on medicines across health communities;
> - supporting prescribers to follow guidance published by professional regulatory bodies in relation to medicines and prescribing (NICE, 2014).

pharmacology, along with specific facts and details about many available medicines. Though it is a national formulary, it nevertheless also includes entries for some medicines which are *not* available under the NHS and must be prescribed and/or purchased privately. A symbol clearly denotes such drugs in their entry.

It is used by healthcare professionals as a reference for correct dosage, indication, inter-actions and side-effects of drugs. Information on drugs is drawn from the manufacturers' product literature, medical and pharmaceutical literature, regulatory authorities and profes-sional bodies. Advice is constructed from clinical literature, and reflects, as far as possible, an evaluation of the evidence from diverse sources.

The BNF also takes account of authoritative national guidelines and emerging safety con-cerns. In addition, the Joint Formulary Committee, which oversees the publication and con-tent of the BNF, takes advice on all therapeutic areas from expert clinicians; this ensures that the BNF recommendations are relevant to practice.

Sister publication

The ***British National Formulary for Children*** (**BNFC**), first published September 2005, is published yearly and details the doses and uses of medicines in children from neonates to adolescents (see Chapter 8 on medicines use in special patient groups). To find out more, go to www.bnf.org/about/

The Drug Tariff

The Drug Tariff provides information on what will be paid to contractors for NHS ser-vices including the cost of drugs and appliances supplied against an NHS prescription but also remuneration to NHS contractors such as pharmacies. To find out more see Drug Tariff, 2023, and www.nhsbsa.nhs.uk/pharmacies-gp-practices-and-appliance-contractors/drug-tariff

Perhaps more important to all prescribers is that in the Drug Tariff there is a section (Section XVIIIA), known unofficially as the 'Blacklist', which lists medicines which cannot be prescribed under the NHS.

There is also a short list within the Drug Tariff which shows those medicines that can be prescribed but only under certain circumstances (Section XVIIIB), the details of which go beyond the scope of this short book. However, it would be useful for you as a prescriber to look at this list at some point.

Neither sections XVIIIA nor B are available on the online version of the Drug Tariff, but you can see a hard copy or view a pdf available from the home page or at www.nhsbsa.nhs.uk/sites/default/files/2022-06/Drug%20Tariff%20July%202022.pdf

The *Nurse Prescribers' Formulary* (NPF)

The *Nurse Prescribers' Formulary for Community Practitioners* (NPF) is a list of medicines that can be prescribed by community practitioner nurse prescribers (CPNPs) who have received training specifically to become such prescribers. It is issued within the BNF every two years.

It covers such areas as laxatives, skin preparations, elastic hosiery (for a full list, see a current NPF) and is the approved list for prescribing by community practitioner nurse prescribers, district nurses and specialist public health nurses, including health visitors. In addition to the relatively brief list are all pharmacy medicines sold under the supervision of a pharmacist and marked with a letter P on packets and a number of prescription-only medicines (POMs), such as nystatin oral suspension, enabling nurses to prescribe in areas such as minor injuries, minor ailments, health promotion and palliative care. The CPNP must only prescribe items from the NPF and for the conditions specifically mentioned. For example, for Co-danthramer oral suspension NPF refers the nurse to the monograph in the BNF but adds that the nurse can prescribe this after consultation with a doctor for constipation in palliative care. So there are some restrictions on the use of the preparation within the NPF. There are a number of appliances as well as medicinal products that can be prescribed by the CPNP. These are shown in the Drug Tariff; Part XVII(B) gives the NPF again, including showing where various appliances can be found. The section is called Appliances and reagents (including wound management products) and also appears in the NPF in the BNF. The CPNP can prescribe:

- appliances as listed in Part IXA (including contraceptive devices);
- incontinence appliances as listed in Part IXB;
- stoma appliances and associated products as listed in Part IXC;
- chemical reagents, as listed in Part IXR.

Table 2.1 The areas covered by the NPF

Analgesics	Emollient and barrier	Prevention of neural tube defects
Appliances and reagents for	preparations	Removal of earwax
diabetes	Eye drop dispensers	Stoma appliances
Contraceptives, non-hormonal	Laxatives	Stoma care
Disinfection and cleansing	Local anaesthetics	Urinary catheters and appliances
Drugs for scabies and head lice	Nicotine replacement therapy	
Drugs for the mouth	Other skin conditions	
Drugs for threadworms	Peak flow meters	

Activity 2.1

Look at a current NPF which is in the BNF. In the hard copy it is towards the back or use the link bnf.nice.org/nurse-prescribers-formulary/

What do you think of the list?

Does it cover the areas with which you are dealing?

Which of the included items are you familiar with and which, if any, have you used or recommended?

These are for community practitioners who have completed the necessary training – not supplementary or independent nurse prescribers.

There is no right or wrong answer here; it is what you think about the list and whether you think it adequate for CPNPs to practice effectively.

The *Electronic Medicines Compendium* (EMC)

The Data Sheet Compendium, as it was known, was a hard copy book containing all of the data sheets, now called summaries of product characteristics (SmPC) for all licensed medicines in the UK. The EMC is, as you can imagine, much easier to handle. The EMC is the most up-to-date, approved and regulated information source on medicines and patient information for licensed drugs. As a healthcare professional you can look at the summary of product characteristics (SmPC) for any licensed drug in the UK. The structure of the entries consistent throughout, giving more detail than the BNF. As this is an important source, the next activity will give you an opportunity to look at it if you haven't already (EMC, 2023).

Activity 2.1

Go to www.medicines.org.uk/emc (EMC, 2023) and look at the front home page. The first thing you see is:

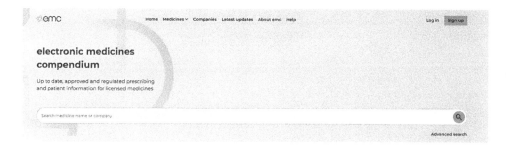

Figure 2.1 EMC home page

© Datapharm and reproduced with kind permission

At the top of the page are tabs you can look at: for example, under the Medicines tab you can see discontinued medicines, which could be useful.

You do not need to register if you are only wishing to look at specific medicines as the SmPC (accessible to healthcare professional) or the patient information leaflet (PIL). Type in the name of the medicine you wish to look at and don't forget to press the magnifying glass symbol. Next you can view the latest updates on this front page.

Latest updates

Spikevax bivalent Original/Omicron BA.4-5 25 micrograms/25 micrograms dispersion for injection
Active ingredients/generics: elasomeran, davesomeran

Moderna Biotech UK Ltd new

Spikevax bivalent Original/Omicron BA.4-5 (50 micrograms/50 micrograms)/mL dispersion for injection
Active ingredients/generics: elasomeran, davesomeran

Moderna Biotech UK Ltd new

Zejula 100 mg hard capsules
Active ingredients/generics: niraparib tosylate monohydrate

GlaxoSmithKline UK updated

More medicines

Figure 2.2 Latest updates

Also on the front page is the link to the Yellow Card reporting system which we will look at in Chapter 9.

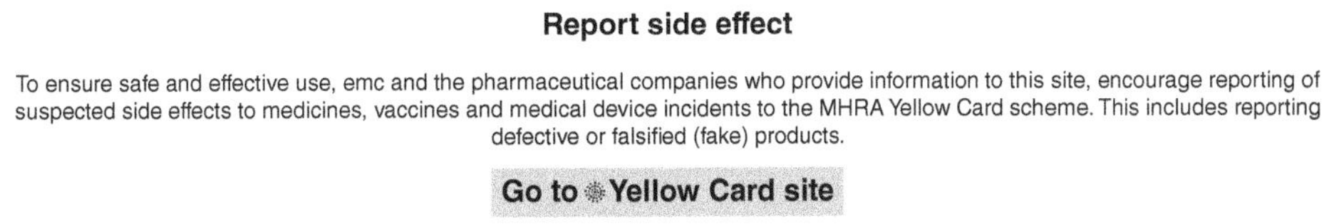

Report side effect

To ensure safe and effective use, emc and the pharmaceutical companies who provide information to this site, encourage reporting of suspected side effects to medicines, vaccines and medical device incidents to the MHRA Yellow Card scheme. This includes reporting defective or falsified (fake) products.

Go to ❋Yellow Card site

Figure 2.3 Yellow Card reporting system

Now search for Perindopril erbumine 8mg tablets by typing the name perindopril in the search box and selecting the correct one. Press the magnifying glass symbol.

You will see:

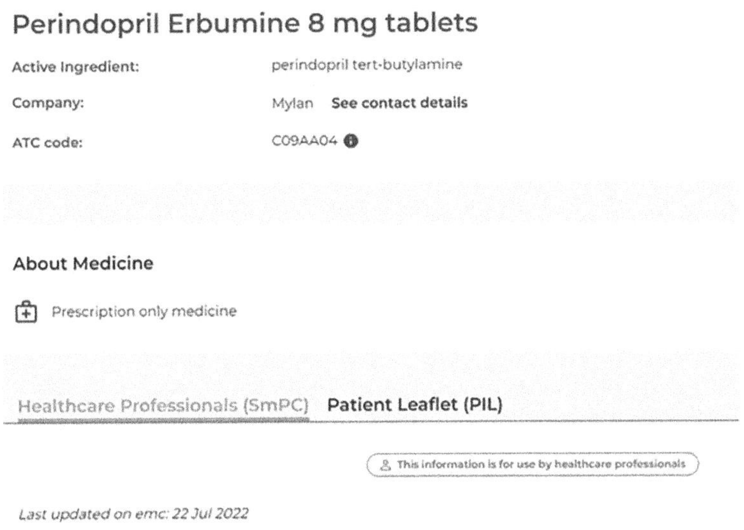

Perindopril Erbumine 8 mg tablets

Active Ingredient:	perindopril tert-butylamine
Company:	Mylan **See contact details**
ATC code:	C09AA04 ⓘ

About Medicine

⊞ Prescription only medicine

Healthcare Professionals (SmPC)   **Patient Leaflet (PIL)**

⚬ This information is for use by healthcare professionals

Last updated on emc: 22 Jul 2022

Figure 2.4 Perindopril erbumine

(Datapharm Perindopril erbumine 8mg tablets showing access to the SmPC and the PIL)

Looking at the SmPC, the structure is the same for all medicines within the EMC; you will need to expand the part of the entry you are interested in. For example, if you expand Section 4, Clinical particulars, you see there are nine further sections.

You can further expand each of these subdivisions such as contraindications or undesirable effects.

Looking specifically at undesirable effects, this gives an initial summary and then lists any reported undesirable effect using an agreed frequency set of definitions.

4. Clinical particulars

4.1 Therapeutic indications

4.2 Posology and method of administration

4.3 Contraindications

4.4 Special warnings and precautions for use

4.5 Interaction with other medicinal products and other forms of interaction

4.6 Fertility, pregnancy and lactation

4.7 Effects on ability to drive and use machines

4.8 Undesirable effects

4.9 Overdose

Figure 2.5   Clinical particulars

Summary of safety profile

The safety profile of perindopril is consistent with the safety profile of ACE inhibitors:

The most frequent adverse events reported in clinical trials and observed with perindopril are: dizziness, headache, paraesthesia, vertigo, visual disturbances, tinnitus, hypotension, cough, dyspnoea, abdominal pain, constipation, diarrhoea, dysgeusia, dyspepsia, nausea, vomiting, pruritis, rash, muscle cramps, and asthenia.

Tabulated list of adverse reactions

The following undesirable effects have been observed during clinical trials and/or post-marketing use with perindopril and ranked under the following frequency:

Very common (≥1/10); Common (≥1/100 to <1/10); Uncommon (≥1/1,000 to <1/100); Rare (≥1/10,000 to <1/1,000); Very rare (<1/10,000); Not known (cannot be estimated from the available data).

Figure 2.6   Initial summary of undesirable effects

© Datapharm and reproduced with kind permission

Note the definitions of Very common, Common, Uncommon, Rare, Very rare and Not known. If a side-effect is said to be Rare that does not mean it may not occur in the patient you are dealing with. In fact, the symbol before each of the definitions is especially important. Take, on the one hand, Very common; the symbol before means 'equal to or more than' 1 in 10. That could mean 10 in 10. Patients may say 1 in 10 means 9 in 10 do not get the side-effect. Draw their attention to the symbol or at least its meaning. On the other hand, the symbol before Very rare is less than 1 in 10,000. The numbers are based on Yellow Card reports of side-effects; those for new drugs may underestimate until more patients have used them. The section then lists all of the reported side-effects and indicates their frequency using the definition above. Also see the section on adverse drug effects and side-effects in Chapter 9 of this book.

> **Activity 2.2**
>
> Now look up any medicine you are familiar with and find the indications and undesirable effects.

As you can see this is a particularly useful source of medicines information. It is up to date and easy to use. The structure for each included medicine is the same.

So, formularies list drugs that you can prescribe; in the case of the Drug Tariff, it shows you which drugs cannot be prescribed on the NHS, or which can only be prescribed under specific circumstances. Formularies are basic lists, but the BNF and the BNFC give guidance on prescribing and each monograph (drug entry) shows what the medicine is for – the indication, when that medicines should be avoided, the contraindications, what advice there is if the patient has hepatic or renal dysfunction, prescribing in pregnancy and prescribing when breast-feeding. The BNF and the BNFC are invaluable to you as a prescriber. The Drug Tariff is more important to pharmacists but still it is worth looking at. The EMC is useful not only for the summary of product characteristics, but also the patient information leaflets that accompany the medicines when they are dispensed, and which are shown in the EMC. It means that during a consultation with a patient you can see what they will be given to read with their prescribed medicine and, if necessary, you can explain certain points.

Frameworks

A framework is a system that guides and supports you when you are dealing with an activity such as prescribing. A competency framework is a structure which describes the competencies (demonstrable knowledge, skills, characteristics, qualities and behaviours) central to a safe and effective performance in a role (RPS, 2021). Looking specifically at prescribing, the National Prescribing Centre (NPC) produced a number of such competency frameworks for the individual groups of prescribers from 2001 onwards.

The first edition, called *Maintaining Competency in Prescribing: An Outline Framework to Help Nurse Prescribers* (NPC, 2001), has a foreword from the then Chief Nursing Office in which she reiterates the ongoing need for nurses to prescribe safely, appropriately and with confidence. Frameworks are the support mechanism needed.

The initial framework was aimed at helping the individual nurse and their managers to identify gaps in knowledge and skills, thus leading to suitable training and development. The framework could also be used by those approved higher education institutions to offer appropriate courses built around the competencies, acting as another layer of support.

The competency framework can also be the structure for continuing professional development (CPD) to ensure if roles change new competencies which may be required can be identified and strengthened.

The first edition, specifically for nurses and not at that time anticipated as being for all prescribers, explained the structure which, although developed over the ten years, has retained its overarching appearance. The NPC suggested that the framework could be used by qualified nurse prescribers as a form of reflection on their day-to-day prescribing, being especially good when used with groups of nurses. Nurses were encouraged to download the framework and adapt or customise it to suit individual needs. The NPC became part of NICE in April 2011.

In 2003 the nurse competency framework was updated and by 2004 other healthcare professions were being accepted onto courses to become supplementary prescribers. The NPC produced individual competency frameworks for pharmacists, optometrists and allied health professionals. These competency frameworks were structured in an equivalent way to the original 2001 nurse competency framework.

The *Competency Framework for All Prescribers*

It was then agreed to produce a single competency framework as all prescribers would need to maintain the same competencies when it came to prescribing. The first framework for all prescribers was published in May 2012, again by the NPC using multidisciplinary expertise. It became clear that 'a common set of competencies underpin prescribing regardless of professional background' (NPC, 2012). The statement in the document said that: 'The single competency framework provides an outline of common prescribing competencies that, if acquired and maintained can help all prescribers to become and remain effective prescribers' (NPC, 2012, p. 4).

The framework can be used by any prescriber at any point in their career. It is not only to guide the prescribing courses, but also for use in CPD and in general sessions with other prescribers.

The proposed use of the framework is shown in **Box 2.2**.

Box 2.2

Uses of the framework include:

1. inform education curricula and relevant accreditation of prescribing programmes;
2. inform the design and delivery of education programmes – for example, through validation of educational sessions (including rationale for need), and as a framework to structure learning and assessment;
3. help healthcare professionals prepare to prescribe and provide the basis for ongoing education and development programmes, and revalidation processes – for example, for use as a framework for a portfolio to demonstrate competency in prescribing;
4. help prescribers identify strengths and areas for development through self-assessment appraisal and as a way of structuring feedback from colleagues;
5. provide professional organisations or specialist groups with a basis for the development of levels of prescribing competency – for example, from recently qualified prescriber through to advanced prescriber;
6. stimulate discussions around prescribing competencies and multidisciplinary skill mix at an organisational level;

7.   inform organisational recruitment processes to help frame questions and benchmark candidates' prescribing experience;

8.   inform the development of organisational systems and processes that support safe, effective prescribing – for example, local clinical governance frameworks.

The current *Competency Framework for All Prescribers*

The framework does suggest that as it does not contain statements that relate to specialist areas of prescribing as it is a competency framework for all prescribers, it must be contextualised to reflect different areas of practice, levels of expertise and settings.

The *Competency Framework* is shown, with permission of the RPS, as Appendix 1 in this book. This framework consolidates the existing profession-specific prescribing frameworks and updates the competencies in order to provide a single common framework that is relevant to doctors, dentists and all other qualified UK prescribers.

The current edition is much more detailed, even as compared to the 2016 one, and has useful notes to help define and explain individual competencies. New ones have been added, as necessary. Prescribing courses across the UK can use this new RPS framework to ensure teaching and practice helps the nurse develop the required competencies.

Appendix 1, which shows the *Competency Framework* (although for the full document please go to www.rpharms.com/resources/frameworks/prescribing-competency-framework/competency-framework) shows that the framework is divided into two domains. Domain 1 covers the consultation (see **Box 2.3**) and Domain 2 prescribing governance (see **Box 2.4**).

Within the two domains there are ten competencies, each with several supporting statements related to the prescriber role showing the activity which the prescriber should demonstrate. Following this are sections on further information which support the prescriber by giving more information about the competency and giving some examples.

Look at the first competency, Assess the patient. Within these there are 14 supporting statements all related to the assessment of the patient. The further information on these supporting statements shows such things as having an appropriate setting for the consultation, using appropriate language for age etc. and understanding that a clinical assessment includes observations, psychosocial assessments and physical examination. The full ten competencies given in Appendix 1, but are shown here for simplicity.

Box 2.3

Domain 1: The consultation

1.   Assess the patient.
2.   Identify evidence-based treatment options available for clinical decision making.
3.   Present options and reach a shared decision.
4.   Prescribe.
5.   Provide information.
6.   Monitor and review.

Looking at competency 4, Prescribe, there are 14 supporting statements and a further four points of further information.

Box 2.4

Domain 2: Prescribing governance

7. Prescribe safely.
8. Prescribe professionally.
9. Improve prescribing practice.
10. Prescribe as part of a team.

Looking at Competency 7, Prescribe safely, there are eight supporting statements and a further three points of further information for this competency.

Now would be a suitable time to look at Appendix 1 and note the depth and range of competencies required to be a prescriber. Remember this is not just for nurses, it is for *all* prescribers.

Throughout this short book, we will point the reader to the appropriate domain and competency.

Summary

In the UK, formularies exist to specify which drugs are available on the NHS for particular groups of prescribers. The two main reference sources providing this information are the BNF and the Drug Tariff.

A framework is a system that guides and supports you when you are dealing with an activity such as prescribing. A competency framework is a structure which describes the competencies (demonstrable knowledge, skills, characteristics, qualities and behaviours) central to a safe and effective performance in a role.

Formularies and frameworks are there to help and support you in your decisions about prescribing for your patients. Familiarise yourself with those related to your area of prescribing.

References

BNF 2022. *British National Formulary: Key Information on the Selection, Prescribing, Dispensing and Administration of Medicines.* Available at bnf.nice.org.uk/ (accessed December 2022).

BNFC 2023. *British National Formulary for Children: Key Information on the Selection, Prescribing, Dispensing and Administration of Medicines.* London: BMJ Group.

Electronic Medicines Compendium. 2023. *Datapharm Perindopril Erbumine 8mg tablets.* (Updated July 2022) Available at https://www.medicines.org.uk/emc/product/4391 (Accessed April 2023). Drug Tariff 2023. Available at faq.nhsbsa.nhs.uk/knowledgebase/article/KA-01493/en-us (accessed December 2022).

EMC 2023. *Electronic Medicines Compendium.* Available at www.medicines.org.uk/emc (accessed December 2022).

Medicinal Products: Prescription By Nurses Etc. Act 1992 (C. 28). [online] London: HMSO. Available at www.legislation.gov.uk/ukpga/1992/28 (accessed 12 May 2023).

Medicines Act 1968 (C. 67). [online] London: HMSO. Available at www.legislation.gov.uk/ukpga/1968/67/contents (accessed 12 May 2023).

NICE 2014. *Medicines Practice Guideline: Developing and Updating Local Formularies.* 14 March. Updated 28 October 2015. Available at www.nice.org.uk/guidance/mpg1 (accessed December 2022).

NPC 2001. *Maintaining Competency in Prescribing: An Outline Framework to Help Nurse Prescribers.* 1st ed. Liverpool: NPC.

NPC 2012. *A Single Competency Framework for All Prescribers.* Liverpool: NPC.

NPF 2022. *Nurse Prescribers' Formulary.* Available at bnf.nice.org.uk/nurse-prescribers-formulary (accessed December 2022).

RPS 2021. *A Competency Framework for All Prescribers.* Available at www.rpharms.com/resources/frameworks/prescribing-competency-framework/competency-framework (accessed 12 May 2023).

3

The Consultation, Diagnostic Processes, Differential Diagnosis and Influences on Prescribing

Melanie McGinlay and Barry Strickland-Hodge

Chapter summary

In this chapter we discuss what good consultation skills are, including actively listening, using positive body language, asking open questions, remaining non-judgemental and exploring patients' ideas, concerns and expectations.

- We explore the patient's and carer's understanding of the outcome of the consultation by summarising necessary, questioning and further explaining.
- We support the diagnostic process by discussing various possibilities (differential diagnosis) and explain the factors that might unduly influence prescribing such as the potential influence of the pharmaceutical industry.
- We will show the competencies that are covered from the *Competency Framework for All Prescribers* (RPS, 2021).

Introduction

A consultation is an opportunity for a patient and health professional to undertake a meeting reliant on discussion and collaboration (Moulton, 2016). While consultation skills can be seen as the tools used to conduct the interaction, in relation to prescribing, there is an expectation that the clinical consultation process incorporates some form of history-taking (medication and medical), assessment, diagnosis, treatment planning and follow-up (Moulton, 2016).

NHS England as part of the *NHS Long Term Plan* (NHS England, 2019) proposes that both patient and health professional are experts during a consultation. There is vast emphasis on the notion of personalised care and shared decision-making, with the endeavour to recognise the bespoke needs of individuals. There is added consideration that patients or their carer bring insight into a patient's values and preferences adjunct to expert knowledge of their illness experience, while the healthcare professional brings their expert knowledge of human pathology and treatment options (Bond et al., 2012). NHS England (2019) also recognises that both patients and healthcare professionals have a role to play in managing consultation expectations with the insight they bring.

Consultation skills

There are a vast number of communication skills required to undertake an effective consultation and such skills can include active listening and questioning, information exchange, non-verbal communication cues, reasoning and the ability to be adaptable and responsive to change. These skills are viewed as paramount in enabling the drawing out of information for diagnostic reasoning and to help formulate a safe and effective plan (Silverman et al., 2008). It is important that practitioners are able to identify and respond to cues as part of the information-gathering phase of the consultation. Such cues can be something the patient says or demonstrates. Non-verbal cues can, debatably, be unconscious signals offered by the patient about what they are potentially thinking and feeling, including facial expressions, tone of voice and body language. Despite these invaluable cues often being thought of as a means of guiding a practitioner to formulate a diagnosis, Silverman et al. (2008) suggest that such cues have a tendency to be routinely overlooked.

Communication skills are commonly adjunct to competence in physical assessment and examination. For some, such skills are a routine part of a consultation and attribute to determining the nature of symptoms – for example, observation and inspection for pathogenomic signs. A carefully conducted consultation has the potential to refine the diagnostic process, prevent unnecessary diagnostic testing and aid a positive relationship between patient and health professional that is built on trust (Moulton, 2016).

Box 3.1

Summary of essential communication skills

Skill	Approach
Active listening skills	Summarise patient's comments, provide feedback, use non-verbal cues to show attention
Questioning skills	Open questions to elicit information Closed question when enough information has been obtained and to close consultation
Giving information	Offer/signpost supportive literature from reputable sources
Non-verbal communication skills	Be mindful of facial expressions and body language in response to the information a patient provides 'Neutrally responsive'
Reasoning skills	Ability to gather appropriate information, interpret and then apply it both in diagnosis and management
Adaptable/responsive to change	Responsive to factors that can influence the consultations e.g., challenging patient, environment

In using the above skills, it is important to remember they have the potential to influence the relationship you develop with the patient during the allotted time. It is also important that they are not used to confuse or mislead the patients to your own agenda as a health professional. Look at some of the example sentences below, these are some of the most commonly used phrases which you are encouraged to avoid

'You have not been having any adverse effects to the medication.'
'You are not having any problems with taking the medication.'

With verbal cues, be mindful to take into consideration tone of voice and personal attitudes to avoid seeming judgemental or frustrated with responses, but also be sure to avoid talking over patients and finishing their sentences. This principle also applies to non-verbal cues – for example, distance, appropriate eye contact and avoiding looking distracted or bored, nodding throughout the consultation and not at the points where you agree or understand what is being said.

Consultation models

Consultation models are commonly used to add structure to a clinical consultation to help avoid the consultation from deteriorating into what can be perceived as disarray and subsequent dysfunction, potentially leading to an ineffectual outcome (Denness, 2013).

The main goal of this approach is to obtain a biomedical (disease) perspective with the patient (illness perspective) as mentioned earlier. This style is then used within the context of a patient's medical, personal and social history. The differing components of such models become apparent where some place greater emphasis on the diagnostic process in contrast to others who focus more on discovering patient priorities.

Although not an exhaustive list, below are some examples of the most popular consultation models to date.

Traditional medical model (Silverman, 2014, p. 459):

a. presenting complaint
b. history of presenting complaint
c. past medical history
d. family history
e. social history
f. drug and allergy history
g. systems review.

Byrne–Long model (1976): This model structures through six steps, which include forming a rapport with a patient, attempting to reveal the reasons for patient attendance, examination, consideration of the problem, formulation of a plan and closing the consultation. Although a highly logical model, which potentially could help health professionals keep to time constraints, the term 'doctor' is used throughout, which can be deemed as paternalistic with the risk of allowing little room for collaboration and shared decision-making – all arguably not in keeping with modern healthcare agenda.

Five-stage model (Neighbour, 1987): This model establishes the consultation by focusing on five key components: connecting, summarising, handover, safety-netting and housekeeping. Neighbour's model can seem well structured and easy to follow while remaining patient-centred, enabling substantial handover of responsibility back to the patient, in keeping with patient's taking responsibility for their own health.

Calgary–Cambridge model (1996): Focusing on providing structure and building the patient–health professional relationship, the Calgary–Cambridge model again is built upon a five-step approach which includes initiating the session, gathering information, physical examination, explanation and planning and closing the session. Unique to this model is that these five steps are under-pinned by 71 micro-skills. Furthermore, it includes the 'triaxial' of health and social care through incorporating physical, psychological and social factors into the template, allowing for a more holistic assessment. Although this model can be perceived as task-orientated and time-consuming, with some elements leaning towards a paternalistic approach, it does successfully help promote a more targeted conversational exchange with a patient-centred method (Main et al., 2010).

BARD (2006): The model puts forwards four prospects for analysis which include behaviours within the consultation, aims of the consultation, the room itself – that is, the consultation environment – and, lastly, the dialogue between patient and practitioner. There is notable simplicity to this model, especially in contrast to the extensive Calgary–Cambridge model, but with this simplicity comes potential risk of paternalistic traits from the health professional (Warren, 2006).

Health belief model: Ideas, concerns and expectations (ICE) (1975): The health belief model is a popular model and used widely as a template for today's health strategy. Much like the Calgary–Cambridge model it proposes an understanding of the patient's perspective and their own health agenda. The abbreviation ICE is derived from a patient's ideas, concerns and expectations. Looking at the subtopics, one can see how such a model could be perceived as more effective at predicting health behaviour and picking up cues during a consultation, while exploring patient anxieties.

Negotiation and care planning

A key part of the consultation is establishing the aim of prescribing and managing expectations of both the patient and health professional (NHS England, 2019). These can be considered as therapeutic objectives that enable a clear purpose of prescribing being identified. Highlighted below are six established aims of prescribing that can be considered during the consultation.

a. **Curative:** Intent of fully resolving an illness and the goal of returning the patient to their status of health before the illness occurred, e.g., antibiotics or chemotherapy.
b. **Symptomatic relief:** Treating the symptoms of an illness/disease without necessarily resolving the underlying problem, e.g., analgesics, steroids or diuretics.
c. **Disease modifying:** Reducing progression of a chronic condition; ACE inhibitors, Tecfidera (dimethyl fumarate) or Methotrexate.
d. **Empirical:** Medication prescribed based on clinical experience prior to confirmation of medical diagnosis; broad spectrum antibiotics.
e. **Tactical:** Prescribing to gain time while collecting information to form a diagnosis; inhalers or antidepressants.
f. **Preventative/prophylactic:** To minimise the risk of symptom/disease occurrence; statins or anticoagulants.

(Cited in Bradbury and Strickland-Hodge, 2014)

For examples of each of these six aims and for a more detailed discussion of the consultation including suggested questions to help elicit responses and more on communication as part of the consultation, see Bradbury and Strickland-Hodge (2014).

Closing the consultation and record keeping

Competency 6 of the *Competency Framework for All Prescribers* (RPS, 2021) is Monitor and review; there are four supporting statements: 6.1. Establishes and maintains a plan for reviewing the patient's treatment, 6.2. Establishes and maintains a plan to monitor the effectiveness of treatment and potential unwanted effects, 6.3. Adapts the management plan in response to ongoing monitoring and review of the patient's condition and preferences and 6.4. Recognises and reports suspected adverse events to medicines and medical devices using appropriate reporting systems.

So, although the consultation may be over as the patient leaves, there is still much to do around follow-up after a treatment plan has been developed and agreed. In the further information to the competency, it says a plan for reviewing includes safety-netting appropriate follow-up or referral. It may be possible and useful to suggest a timescale for review. In Competency 4, Prescribe, one of the supporting statements is 'documents accurate, legible and contemporaneous clinical records'. This is not only for you, of course, but also for any other prescriber who may need to deal with the patient in the future.

Differential diagnosis and the diagnostic process

The supporting statements around Competency 1, Assess the patient, all deal with the consultation and decision-making. Statement 1.11 is 'makes, confirms or understands, and documents the working or final diagnosis by systematically considering the various possibilities (differential diagnosis)'. This will be considered in this section.

The consultation consists of information-gathering from the patient's record; understanding the reason for the patient's current visit; a physical examination if necessary; and ordering any diagnostic testing in house or through the laboratory services as necessary. All are potentially necessary to create a working or differential diagnosis. The differential diagnosis is where you, as the prescriber and healthcare professional, weigh up the likelihood of one condition over another (Llewelyn et al., 2014). It is then important that you explain the diagnosis and communicate to the patient and/or carer a treatment plan and any necessary ongoing monitoring.

Shared decision-making between you and the patient or their carer is essential for the relationship to be concordant. This is a joint process where you work together to reach a decision about the patient's care (NICE, 2021). The *Competency Framework for All Prescribers* (RPS, 2021) emphasises the importance of maintaining a patient-centred approach when speaking to patients/carers while maintaining confidentiality. In the framework, Competency 3 is Present options and reach a shared decision; the first supporting statement is: 'Actively involves and works with the patient/carer to make informed choices and agree a plan that respects the patient's/carer's preferences', with the further information stating, 'preferences include patient's/carer's right to decline or limit treatment'. This may be a difficult position for you when you have gone through the consultation taking account of all the relevant facts and may have obtained test results, to hear the patient decline your recommendation, but that is their decision and right.

Using the patient's previous experience is a key part of the information-gathering stage to support the differential and final diagnosis.

There are many decision-making models and tools used in practice to help you. Some break down the overall process into a number of structured steps or stages which can help you to use a step-by-step approach to formulate a decision.

Activity 3.1

Think about the steps you need to consider when first making a differential diagnosis and firming this up into a diagnosis and potential treatment regime. The steps in **Answer 3.1** are the basic ones often used, but you may wish to look for other tools – particularly when you are starting out as a new prescriber.

Answer 3.1

Possible overall steps to take you from differential diagnosis to diagnosis.

1. First, identify the problem through talking to and listening to the patient. Leave space for the patient to add anything they think is relevant. Ask questions about the patient's symptoms.
2. At the same time review the patient's medical history as this may have an important impact on your decision-making.
3. If necessary, perform a physical examination which will help to create a 'differential diagnosis' – in other words a range of possibilities at this stage. It may, of course, be obvious, but you need to confirm your decision.
4. Again, if necessary, order any relevant additional tests.
5. Once the results are in, they need to be reviewed in light of what you have already gathered about the presenting symptoms.

Finally, you can make a diagnosis and consider treatment or referral.

Influencing your decision-making

There are many factors that could influence your decision-making – for example, clinical guidelines or patient preferences, as well as the environment in which the consultation takes place. It is important to note that you, as the decision-maker, may have a personal bias subsequent to a previous experience. The combination of intuition based on your previous experience and the patient in front of you and analytic methods such as the physical examination and any laboratory tests undertaken allows you to help create the differential diagnosis, irrespective of your level of experience.

There may be what you might call potential 'risks of judgement errors' such as misperceiving, misreading or misinterpreting information (Kahneman et al., 1982). It can happen at any time once you have an idea in your head about the condition or when using mental short-cuts based on previous experience which may not be exactly the same as the situation you are observing. An example in psychiatry could be the misinterpretation of cognitive decline with an elderly patient taking benzodiazepines. Drug elimination is less efficient in older people and drugs can have prolonged or greater effects in extremes of age. This is important with, for example, benzodiazepines as there can be an accumulation even if the dose is maintained at normal levels. Benzodiazepines can produce more confusion but less sedation in elderly people and any confusion could be misattributed to age-related memory impairment rather than to the drug accumulation.

The influences on prescribing

There are many ways you as a prescriber can be influenced. The most important thing to remember is that evidence-based information is available to you. We are all susceptible – a worthwhile statement with which to begin a short section on influences on prescribing. What might influence you to prescribe a certain medicine? List those you feel are important and check **Box 3.2** at the end to see if you missed any or have considered others.

In the *Competency Framework for All Prescribers* (RPS, 2021), influence is considered and is part of Competency 8, Prescribe professionally; under the supporting statement 8.5, it says 'Recognises and responds to factors that might influence prescribing'. Factors include interactions with pharmaceutical industry, media, patients/carers, colleagues, cognitive bias, financial gain, prescribing incentive schemes, switches and targets.

Influences that could affect your prescribing have been researched for many years and continue to create interest and original research papers (Carter et al., 2021). If a patient has a bad experience or develops a side-effect to a medicine you have prescribed, then this may have an influence on your future prescribing of that medicine.

Recent research has tended to be about influences on prescribing in general practice. Of course, the prescribers in general practice can be a varied group of healthcare professionals – for example, doctors, prescribing nurses, prescribing pharmacists and, in some cases, other prescribing healthcare professionals.

A major influence on all prescribers in general practice will be the quality and outcomes frameworks (QOF) (see **Box 3.3** for an explanation of this). Nationally, there are NICE guidelines which are influential in a number of ways including the choice of medication for particular conditions. Integrated care boards (ICBs) replaced clinical commissioning groups (CCGs) in the NHS in England from 1 July 2022. They may make recommendations or even offer incentives to prescribe in a certain way to increase the amount of generic prescribing. National guidelines can be linked to other local initiatives to influence the prescriber as to what is prescribed.

If you have used online prescribing support tools such as ScriptSwitch, which can be used to promote NICE guidelines, you will be aware of the support they give as you prescribe. It is a computer program that interacts with GP clinical systems and operates at the point of prescribing to promote rational prescribing choices.

If a practice has practice meetings such guidelines, the impact of QOF can be discussed among the staff, again to promote evidence-based, rational prescribing choices.

Another influence is your own professional background education, experience and beliefs which can impact on what you choose for a patient once the diagnosis has been agreed. You might call this habit; you have prescribed for this condition so often but you need to keep up to date and ensure the treatment you have used before is still the best.

It is possible that the ICB has a formulary which it would anticipate you would follow; adherence to this can of be reviewed by the ICB. Prescribing analysis and cost (PACT) data has been available since the end of the 1980s and it analyses every prescription that is dispensed. Advisers may come in and discuss your prescribing habits or the practice's prescribing habits and that may have an influence.

As a prescriber you will be expected to work within your sphere of competence – your scope of practice – so that you only prescribe within your competence level. Over time, of course, you will gain experience; you will note that certain things that you have prescribed were particularly useful or successful and you may continue them. Much will have to do with your confidence, experience and your ability to undertake CPD.

You might argue that where you practise will have an influence. For example, in an affluent area patients may be able and willing to buy their medication if available over the counter. In a more deprived area, you may be prescribing those same things. Also, in an affluent area you may have patients who make more demands.

In some GP practices there are staff who specialise and it may be from them you will get advice and support for your prescribing choices. This informal type of learning will develop over time and will affect your choices.

We come to the area of the pharmaceutical company, which was, in my view, much more influential ten or 20 years ago. It is not just the company representative who may visit or offer you lunch or host a meeting or even host educational events. There are adverts even in professional and free journals.

In general practice the knowledge and experience from each professional group in the practice such as nurses, pharmacists, GPs and other healthcare professionals will help develop and shape your prescribing within that practice.

You can see there are many potential influences on your prescribing

If you look at secondary care formularies, guidelines and the medicines committee will all have an influence on what is prescribed in that hospital. Adherence to the formularies will be expected. The pharmaceutical industry can again have an influence in various ways. Costs in hospital may be kept artificially low but when the patient returns to primary care and receives the recommended medication at full cost, the hospital may be having an influence on your prescribing. If you have a practice-based pharmacist, they are there to ask questions as well as do their own work; they can support you in terms of medicines optimisation and review.

So, in summary, we have national and local guidelines from the Royal colleges, from NICE and from ICBs.

Patients themselves will have an influence, based on their experiences in the past. Primary care networks (PCNs), where groups of practices work together, may also have an influence on the overall choice of medicines for particular conditions.

You are an influence on your own prescribing – your own experiences, your background your knowledge or competencies. These will all dictate, to some extent, what you will prescribe in the early days of being a prescriber; you will take much more advice from your colleagues. As you gain experience you will be the one who will give advice.

As was mentioned earlier, we are all susceptible; be on your guard and do not be swayed by anything other than evidence, discussions with experts and your own reading and CPD.

Box 3.2

Potential influences on your prescribing are:

1. you, your background, experience, education and beliefs;
2. the patient and where you practice;
3. colleagues, experts you may know, specialists where you practice;
4. the practice, practice meetings, QOF;
5. national and local guidelines, NICE etc.;
6. integrated care boards (ICBs) formerly clinical commissioning groups (CCGs);
7. hospital requests for your patients;
8. online prescribing support tools such as ScriptSwitch;
9. the pharmaceutical industry, company representative, adverts, meetings, EMC;
10. continuing professional development (CPD).

Box 3.3

The objective of the quality and outcomes framework (QOF) is to improve the service patients are given by rewarding practices for the quality of care they provide to their patients, based on several indicators across a range of key areas of clinical care and public health. Measures, called indicators, are agreed as part of the GP contract negotiations every year. These indicators have points attached that are given to GP practices based on how they are doing against these measures.

The indicators include: management of some of the most common chronic conditions – for example, asthma and diabetes; management of major public health concerns – for example, smoking and obesity; and providing preventative services such as screening or blood pressure checks.

In the 2021–2 QOF there are, for example, new vaccination and immunisation indicators and a new indicator for cancer care (NHS Digital Data Publications, 2022).

Summary

A consultation is an opportunity for a patient and health professional to undertake a meeting reliant on discussion and collaboration. Consultation skills can include active listening and questioning, information exchange, non-verbal communication cues, reasoning and the ability to be adaptable and responsive to change. There are various models to guide you and to add structure to a clinical consultation. Remember, decision-making is a shared action that demands engaging patients as experts in their own health. Once the diagnosis or the management decisions have been concluded, it is then important that you explain the diagnosis and communicate to the patient and/or carer, a treatment plan and any necessary ongoing monitoring. There are many factors that could influence your decision-making – for example, clinical guidelines or patient preferences, as well as the environment in which the consultation takes place. Be aware that anyone can be influenced.

References

Bond, C., Blenkinsopp, A. and Raynor, D.K. 2012. Prescribing and partnership with patients. *British Journal of Clinical Pharmacology.* **74**(4), pp. 581–8.

Bradbury, H. and Strickland-Hodge, B. 2014. *Practical Prescribing for Medical Students.* London: Sage.

Carter, M., Chapman, S. and Watson, M.C. 2021. Multiplicity and complexity: A qualitative exploration of influences on prescribing in UK general practice. *BMJ Open.* Available at strathprints.strath.ac.uk/75414/1/Carter_etal_BMJO_2021_Multiplicity_complexity_qualitative_exploration_influences_prescribing_UK.pdf (accessed December 2022).

Denness, C. 2013. What are consultation models for? *InnovAiT: Education and Inspiration for General Practice.* **6**(9), pp. 592–9.

Hacking, I. 2001. *An Introduction to Probability, and Deductive Logic.* Cambridge: Cambridge University Press.

ICE Model 2 Revisiting Models of the Consultation IN Med Care. Becker, M.H. and Maiman, L.A., 1975. Sociobehavioral determinants of compliance with health and medical care recommendations. Medical care, pp.10–24.

Kahneman, D., Slovic, P. and Tversky, A. 1982 *Judgement Under Uncertainty: Heuristics and Biases.* Cambridge: Cambridge University Press.

Kurtz, S.M. and Silverman, J.S., 1996. The Calgary-Cambridge Observation Guides: an aid to defining the curriculum and organising the teaching in Communication Training Programmes. Med Education, 30, pp. 83–9

Llewelyn H., Aun Ang H., Lewis K. and Al-Abdullah, A. 2014. *Oxford Handbook of Clinical Diagnosis.* 3rd ed. Oxford: Oxford University Press.

Main, C.J., Buchbinder., R, Porcheret, M. and Foster, N. 2010. Addressing patient beliefs and expectations in the consultation. *Best Practice and Research: Clinical Rheumatology.* **24**(2), pp. 219–25.

Mehay, R. 2012. *The Essential Handbook for GP Training and Education.* 1st ed. London: Radcliffe.

Moulton, L. 2016. *The Naked Consultation: A Practical Guide to Primary Care Consultation Skills.* 2nd ed. Boca Raton, FL: CRCPress.

Neighbour, R. 1987. *The Inner Consultation.* Oxford: Radcliffe Medical Press.

NHS Digital Data Publications 2022. *Quality and Outcomes Framework, 2021–2022.* Available at digital.nhs.uk/data-and-information/publications/statistical/quality-and-outcomes-framework-achievement-prevalence-and-exceptions-data/2021-22 (accessed 15 May 2023).

NHS England 2019. *The NHS Long Term Plan.* Available at: www.longtermplan.nhs.uk/wp-content/uploads/2019/08/nhs-long-term-plan-version-1.2.pdf (accessed 26 September 2022).

NICE 2021. *Shared decision making.* Available at www.nice.org.uk/about/what-we-do/our-programmes/nice-guidance/nice-guidelines/shared-decision-making (accessed June 2021).

RPS 2021. *A Competency Framework for All Prescribers.* Available at www.rpharms.com/resources/frameworks/prescribers-competency-framework (accessed 12 May 2023).

Silverman J., Kurtz S. and Draper J. 2008. *Skills for Communicating with Patients.* Oxford: Radcliffe Medical Press.

Silverman D. 2014. Interpreting qualitative data methods for analysing talk 3rd edition. London: Sage publications.

Warren, E. 2006. *BARD in the Practice: A Guide for Family Doctors to Consult Efficiently, Effectively and Happily.* Oxford: Radcliffe Medical Press.

4

Putting Shared Decision-making into Practice

Rebecca Dickinson, Melanie McGinlay, Helen Bradbury and Sue Alldred

Chapter summary

This chapter discusses working with patients and carers about medicine-taking – for example, ensuring patients and carers understand and are able to adhere to their medicine.

- We explore how to communicate risk, benefits and consequences and discuss patient decision aids.
- This chapter will explore the concepts of risk, benefit and uncertainty, concepts that are central to informed consent and decision-making.
- Different approaches of communicating risk of harm, likelihood of benefit and uncertainty associated with medicine-taking are examined to help you develop an awareness of essential methods of risk communication in order to optimise understanding about medicines and to support informed decision-making.
- This chapter builds on the discussion about adverse drug reactions and side-effects which you will need to manage to reduce risk to the patient.
- It goes on to explore team working and understanding of the roles of different members of the multidisciplinary team (MDT). MDTs in general practice are included here. We consider working collaboratively as part of that team to ensure a safe and effective transfer and continuity of care process is developed.

Introduction

The *Competency Framework for All Prescribers* (RPS, 2021) identifies a number of prescribing areas where there may be associated risk; it is your duty of care, as the nurse prescriber, to minimise these potential risks. Risks can come in several forms which are identified in the RPS framework supporting statements – for example, 2.3, the risks and benefits to the patient of taking or not taking a medicine or treatment, or 4.6, the need to prescribe appropriate quantities of medicine and at appropriate intervals necessary to reduce the risk of unnecessary waste and 4.7, recognising the potential misuse of medicines and minimising the risk by using appropriate processes.

Duty of care

As a nurse and as a nurse prescriber you must be aware of your duty of care when communicating information about medicines to patients. Another of the RPS framework supporting statements which includes this potential risk is 3.3, explaining the material risks and benefits, and rationale behind your chosen management options (*which will include your prescribing decisions*) in a way the patient or carer understands, so that they can make an informed choice. As well as providing information about the potential for risk of harm you should also ensure patients have information about the likelihood of benefit of the treatments prescribed to them in order to promote informed consent (Blalock et al., 2019).

Montgomery v Lanarkshire (2015) is a landmark case that sets the standards for informed consent and the disclosure of risk associated with medical interventions (Chan et al., 2017). The case was brought by Mrs Montgomery, who experienced a traumatic birth that resulted in long-term harm to her baby. Mrs Montgomery successfully argued that she had experienced negligent care due to the lack of disclosure of a rare risk of shoulder dystocia associated with her clinical presentation; she asserted that had she known about the chance of this risk she would have made a different decision about her care, thus mitigating the risk of harm to her baby (Montgomery v Lanarkshire Health Board, 2015).

The outcome of this case sets out a duty of care to communicate about risk to patients with the general principle that clinicians should communicate information that:

> a reasonable person in the patient's position would be likely to attach significance to the risk, or the doctor is or should reasonably be aware that the particular patient would be likely to attach significance to it. (Montgomery v Lanarkshire Health Board, 2015; Chan et al., 2017)

Nurse prescribers must be aware of this duty of care when communicating about medicines to patients. As well as providing information about the potential for risk of harm, nurse prescribers should also ensure patients have information about the likelihood of benefit of the treatments prescribed to them in order to promote informed consent (Blalock et al., 2019).

Communicating risks, benefits and uncertainty about medicines to patients

Risk of harm

Risk can be defined as a potential harmful outcome that can occur with a known or unknown probability (Berry, 2004). The risk of harm associated with medicine-taking typically refers to the likelihood of experiencing a side-effect associated with a treatment (Dickinson, 2014). All medicines can cause harm and the frequency and severity to which a person might experience a side-effect may vary from drug to drug.

Likelihood of benefit

Benefit information is less readily available for prescribers to access as compared to side-effect information. However, its provision is equally important in order to support people making judgements and decisions about the trade-off associated with medicines (Dickinson, 2014). There is no agreed definition of what benefit information encompasses, but it tends to refer to information about how the medicine works and how effective it is.

The MHRA (2005) introduced the concept of benefit information in medicines information, describing it as additional material that describes the positive effects of taking a medicine and refers to several key points it might include, such as:

- why it is important to treat the disease and what the likely clinical outcome would be if the disease remained untreated;
- whether the treatment is for short term or for chronic use;
- whether the medicine is being used to treat the underlying disease (i.e., curative) or for control of symptoms. If the latter, which symptoms will be controlled and how long the effects will last;
- whether the effects will last after the medication is stopped;
- where the medicine is used to treat two or more discrete indications, all should be succinctly described as above;
- where to obtain more information on the condition.

Uncertainty

Uncertainty associated with healthcare conditions and interventions is a complex concept. Uncertainty can be associated with a lack of knowledge or information about a particular diagnosis, prognosis or treatment option. Mishel (1990) defines uncertainty in illness as 'the inability to determine the meaning of illness related events'. As nurses you will be aware of challenges with diagnosing illness and disease due to ambiguous, complex or unpredictable symptoms (Politi et al., 2007). Uncertainty can also be associated with a lack of information about a particular condition or treatment, or because of poor/low quality associated with evidence (Van der Bles et al., 2019; Politi et al., 2007). As evidence-based practitioners you should be aware of how the hierarchy of evidence can be used to understand the efficacy of drugs, with data from well-designed meta-analyses typically more reliable than data from studies with weaker methodologies and study designs.

The impact of communicating risk, benefit and uncertainty information

It is essential that you as a prescriber develop skills in communicating risk, benefit and uncertainty to ensure they meet the legal and ethical requirements of obtaining informed consent (Chan et al., 2017).

This next section will set out some different methods that can be used to support patients to understand more about the risk of harm and likelihood of benefit of the treatments you prescribe.

As a prescriber, you need to be aware that different approaches can have different influences on understanding, emotional responses to information and, ultimately, on medicine-taking behaviour (Van der Bles et al., 2019). It is worth exploring the evidence-base for the different approaches to understand the impacts.

Different approaches to communicating risk, benefit and uncertainty

Verbal and textual approaches

Commonly what people want to know about side-effects include the following:

1. probability
2. severity
3. controllability
4. reversibility
5. time of onset (e.g., whether potential harm usually occurs soon after initiation of therapy or may not arise for many years).

(Bogardus et al., 1999; Blalock et al., 2019)

There is evidence that patients value and want this type of information about their medicines because it can help provide perspective and support decision-making (Knapp et al., 2009; Berry et al., 2002; Berry et al., 2003).

The use of verbal descriptions alone can lead to the overestimation of risk, but this can be mitigated with the inclusion of the numerical descriptors, which has been shown to decrease side-effect expectations and improve medicine adherence. You can easily access this information and use it to support informed decision-making more effectively for patients. It is important to note that patients do not want written medicines information to replace conversations about medicines; however, they do value the inclusion of written information about their medicines (PILs are sometimes the only written information a person receives about their medicines). PILs can be used as an aide memoire to support these discussions with patients to enhance understanding about risks of harm. The use of qualifying verbal statements or descriptors tends to be the most common approach used to describe medicines (Juanchich and Sirota, 2020). It is likely you already use this approach to explain the chance of side-effects or how well a medicine will work to patients using phrases such as around x, roughly x, very likely x, probably x. It denotes a magnitude of effect. This approach tends to be understood by most people and can be reassuring. However, you need to be aware of the potential for patients to overestimate the benefits of their treatments. This is a problem that has been identified in the literature and you should be aware that patients may have unrealistic expectations about the effects of medicines and that they can struggle to understand the magnitude of effects (Hoffmann and Del Mar, 2015; Dickinson et al., 2016).

Numerical depictions

There are many ways to present numerical depictions of risk.

Percentages

This is a commonly used approach to explaining benefits. Many people are experienced with using percentages; however, be aware that not everyone can comprehend or use percentages with ease (Dickinson et al., 2016).

Frequencies

A frequency describes an event, such as a proportion of people with a disease or side-effect, as well as the size of the pre-defined population of interest. There is a significant amount of evidence that this technique can help patients understand the chance of their treatments being effective or resulting in harm more clearly (Akl et al., 2011; Gigerenzer, 2011). There is also good evidence that the use of the technique supports you as a clinician to better understand chance more than, for example, percentages (Gigerenzer, 2011).

Numbers Needed to Treat (NNTs)

A number needed to treat communicates the number of patients that need to be treated to experience an outcome (this might be a side-effect, in which case it would be numbers needed to harm, or a benefit of the treatment). For those that understand this approach, it can lead to a better grasp of treatments effects (Dickinson et al., 2016). There are several textbooks and papers that discuss NNTs such as Ranganathan et al. (2016). An example of how to calculate this is given in the section on calculations in Appendix 3.

Combinations of words and numbers

In practice, as a prescriber you may wish to consider the use of both words and numbers when communicating to patients. This approach is already mandated to communicate about the side-effects of medicines in PILs and can also be accessed in the BNF. There is evidence this approach is useful for patients to understand the magnitude of risk of side-effects.

Another approach is the use of a decision aid. A decision aid is an intervention designed to enhance shared decision-making about a specific clinical decision between patients and clinicians. A decision aid will provide details about options, risks, benefits and uncertainties and ought to be used alongside consultation regarding a decision to support informed choices (Drug and Therapeutics Bulletin, 2013). More information about decision aids is provided later in this chapter.

The communication of information about the uncertainty, the risk of harm and the likelihood of benefit is complex. However, it is essential that you undertake this effectively. Communicating this type of information supports patients with making informed decisions about their medicines. It is essential to develop competence regarding this as you will be expected to be skilled in weighing up the risks and benefits of treatments. There is an expectation you can also explain the material risks and benefits, and rationale behind management options in a way the patient/carer understands; this is now a legal requirement (Chan et al., 2017).

As a prescriber you need to develop your understanding of the different approaches to explaining risk of harm, likelihood of benefit and uncertainty to patients and employ these methods to support better understanding and knowledge about the treatments being prescribed.

Patient decision aids

The *Competency Framework for All Prescribers* (RPS, 2021) includes a number of points and competencies which link to the patient and/or their carer making decisions – in particular, Competency 3, Present options and reach a shared decision, where the supporting statement 3.1 states, 'Actively involves and works with the patient/carer to make informed choices and agree a plan that respects the patient's/carer's preferences'; 3.2: 'Considers and respects patient diversity, background, personal values and beliefs about their health, treatment and medicines, supporting the values of equality and inclusivity, and developing cultural competence'; and 3.3: 'Explains the material risks and benefits, and rationale behind management options in a way the patient/carer understands, so that they can make an informed choice'.

What are patient decision aids?

A patient decision aid is an evidence-based resource designed to help and support patients make decisions when there are choices about different treatments. A decision aid should set out the options, risks and benefits of the recommended treatment pathways (Stacey et al., 2021). They can be really useful devices for you to use with your patient to support you when faced with tricky options about different treatments.

Decision aids should set out the options associated with treatment in a balanced and informative way. The aim of a decision aid is not to influence a patient to choose one treatment over another, but instead to represent the facts about a treatment to a patient in a way that presents a balanced account of the risk of harm with the likelihood of benefit to facilitate patients to make choices that match their values and beliefs (NICE, 2021). A Cochrane systematic review on decision aids explains that: 'People can use decision aids when there is more than one option and neither is clearly better, or when options have benefits and harms that people value differently' (Stacey et al., 2017).

These useful resources can take a number of different formats and may include pamphlets and leaflets, videos or web-based tools. There is a good deal of evidence that patient decision aids can improve patient knowledge and help them feel better informed about what matters most to them (Stacey et al., 2017).

So informed choices are at the centre of your prescribing and will form a major part of your consultation. Decision aids help you and help and support your patient, particularly when decisions about their treatment have options. The decision aid can be useful as a means of structuring a conversation about what the decision entails. It can also be used to promote an in-depth exploration of the choices at hand in partnership with the patient.

Where to find decision aids

You can find a whole range of decision aids for multiple different conditions and health choices from a variety of different organisations. A few examples have been provided in **Box 4.1**.

Box 4.1

NICE – Making decisions about your care (NICE, 2021) includes a range of decisions aids that are relevant to prescribing. These include the following:

- How do I control my blood pressure? Lifestyle options and choice of medicines: patient decision aid.
- Taking a statin to reduce the risk of coronary heart disease and stroke.
- Option grid to help people make decisions about long-term heartburn treatment.
- Bisphosphonates for treating osteoporosis: Decision support from NICE.

Public Health England (although now disbanded) also has a range of decisions aids including the following:

- Making a decision about further treatment for atrial fibrillation.
- Making a decision about open-angle glaucoma.

The Ottawa Hospital Research Institute has undertaken research into the effectiveness of decision aids for decades and has a large repository of decision aids designed to support health decisions about a range of complex health choices. The conditions covered are diverse and include decisions about treatments for acne, angina, atrial fibrillation, depression, various cancers, diabetes, haemorrhoids, menopause, smoking cessation, vaccines and weight control. These can be easily accessed online: decisionaid.ohri.ca/AZlist.html

---

What should a decision aid include?

Ultimately, the aim of a decision aid is to inform patients and support decisions about treatment options; a well-designed decision aid needs to give impartial information in a way that is understandable and which clearly sets out the options associated with the treatment.

NICE (2021) provides a *Standards Framework for Shared-Decision-Making Support Tools* which includes patient decision aids. This document sets out some of the standards decision aids and tools should meet. It is important that key details about the condition and disease need to be set out using accessible, plain and everyday language. This needs to be communicated in a way that accurately represents the impact of the health condition and which sets out the options that are available to the patient. Ideally this should be framed in a patient-focused way, concentrating on what matters to them, rather than on clinical outcomes that might not be relevant to a person's experience of health. You, as the prescriber, should be aware of these and guide your patient as necessary. You may need to explain terms but they should be self-explanatory. Your role, like the decision aid, is to support your patient in making that decision.

As we have mentioned above, numerical data should be used to communicate the options and in ways that are understandable for people with lower levels of numeracy. You can use the section above to reflect on the different approaches to expressing numerical data and identify the best approaches. Numerical information should present the balance between risk of harm and likelihood of benefit.

Decision aids frequently use graphical techniques to present risk and benefits. There are a range of approaches in using graphs to present risk. You may have seen the 'smiley faces' graphs which are commonly useds; these are technically called icon arrays. Other graphical formats can include bar charts, line graphs, risk ladders and pie charts (Stone et al., 2017). Some examples can be seen in the figures.

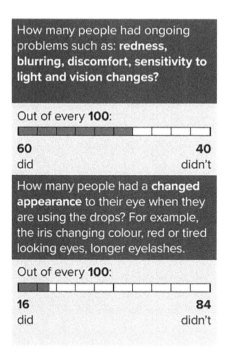

Figure 4.1 An example of a bar chart NHS England

Cardiovascular risk 10% over 10 years: no treatment

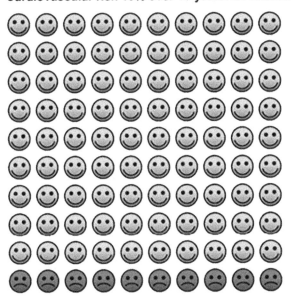

If 100 people at this level of risk take no statin, over 10 years on average:

- 90 people will not develop CHD or have a stroke (the green faces)
- 10 people will develop CHD or have a stroke (the red faces).

Figure 4.2 An example of a 'smiley face' icon array

© www.nice.org.uk/guidance/cg181/resources/patient-decision-aid-pdf-243780159. Reproduced with kind permission © NICE (2014)

Effect of bisphosphonates on the risk of vertebral (spinal) fractures

10 in 100 (10%) baseline risk

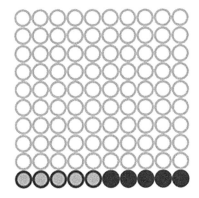

On average, for every 100 people at this baseline risk who have bisphosphonate treatment for at least 3 years, over 10 years:

about 90 people will not have a vertebral fracture and would not have done anyway

about 5 people avoid getting vertebral fractures because they have bisphosphonate treatment

about 5 people get vertebral fractures even though they have bisphosphonate treatment.

Figure 4.3 An example of an icon array

© www.nice.org.uk/guidance/ta464/resources/bisphosphonates-for-treating-osteoporosis-patient-decision-aid-pdf-6896787085. Reproduced with kind permission NICE (2019)

Remember that the use of graphical techniques can also provoke an emotional, affective response in people, similar to the response that can be provided with the use of numerical representations of risk and benefit. Different formats might also be perceived differently by patients, depending upon familiarity and graphical literacy (Oudhoff and Timmermans, 2015). There is no perfect format that meets the needs of all people and you should aim to keep any graphical formats used as clear and simple as possible.

Decision aids should also communicate about the sources of evidence used to support the information provided. The certainty of the evidence and the sources from which it has been derived need to be presented to the patient in an understandable way. You should also make attempts to avoid discrimination and promote equality across the population, so work towards the provision of accessible information (Equality Act, 2010).

Summary of decision aids

To summarise, decisions aids can be a useful device for both patients and prescribers to explore difficult treatment options. As part of your obligation to work with patients in partnership to identify evidence-based treatment options available for clinical decision-making and to present options and reach a shared decision, you will need to succinctly summarise some complex information about treatment options. A decision aid is a device that can assist both you and the patient to understand the options and feel better informed and clearer about what matters most in relation to a complex health decision. There is evidence that decision aids can enhance the accuracy of a patient's expectations of the risks and benefits of treatments and support decision-making that is in line with their values and beliefs (Stacey et al., 2017). The evidence for decision aids is abundant and the research supporting their efficacy is good quality.

You, in your role as a prescriber, should be aware of these useful resources and use them regularly to support shared decision-making about medicines in everyday practice.

Working with others as part of the multidisciplinary team

Multidisciplinary teams (MDTs) are more usually found in hospitals, although primary care is now expanding to include many other healthcare professions such as pharmacists and physiotherapists in one building.

A description of primary care teams is shown below. These too can be seen as MDTs and should be used for their individual skills and specialities. Whether in hospital or primary care, it is important that you are working for the benefit of patients in your care and you are not alone. Always be prepared to ask others for advice and support when needed.

In the *Competency Framework for All Prescribers* (RPS, 2021) a range of competencies are linked to working with others. Competency 10, Prescribe as part of a team, has the supporting statements: 10.1 'Works collaboratively as part of a multidisciplinary team to ensure that the transfer and continuity of care (within and across all care settings) is developed and not compromised'; 10.2 'Establishes relationships with other professionals based on understanding, trust and respect for each other's roles in relation to the patient's care'; 10.3 'Agrees the appropriate level of support and supervision for their role as a pre-scriber'; and 10.4 'Provides support and advice to other prescribers or those involved in administration of medicines where appropriate'. In addition, Competency 1, Assess the patient, has supporting statement 1.14 'Refers to or seeks guidance from another mem-ber of the team, a specialist or appropriate information source when necessary'; Com-petency 4, Prescribe, has supporting statement 4.14 'Effectively and securely communi-cates information to other healthcare professionals involved in the patient's care, when sharing or transferring care and prescribing responsibilities, within and across all care settings'.

As a nurse prescriber you will be one of many healthcare professionals involved in a patient's care. While some of these may form part of the hospital healthcare team, others will be located within primary care or elsewhere. In order that patient care is not compro-mised, it remains incumbent upon every member of the team to collaborate with each other, thus contributing to the MDT, ensuring safe, effective prescribing for patients. With changes in healthcare policy driving the need for MDT working, following on from the NHS *People Plan* (2020), Health Education England (HEE) published a toolkit to help organisations and healthcare professionals to work differently to develop a one-workforce approach to patient care (NHS, 2021). This toolkit provides a useful framework for you and your organisation to use when developing and reviewing MDT working; it identifies six enablers for team working. These are planning and design, skill mix and learning, culture, shared goals and objectives, working across boundaries and communication. Although good leadership in organisations is a key component of successful MDT working, as a nurse prescriber your understanding of these enablers will help you achieve the competencies listed above in the RPS framework (RPS, 2021).

Enablers to working in a multidisciplinary team

When thinking about planning and design it is paramount that the right people, with the right skills and competencies, are brought together in the right place at the right time. This must be based on population needs and shaped by the patients and communities being served (Thorstensen-Woll et al., 2021). Having the patient at the centre should be the focus for all MDTs, regardless of setting, and this means having a shared commitment to personalised care from the perspective of the individual. Ensuring the right skill mix, where roles and tasks are carefully articulated, helps to build shared expectations and awareness of roles and respon-sibilities for specific activities (Baird et al., 2020). There is the potential for MDTs to blur boundaries between roles which could cause anxiety if team members feel their professional identity is threatened. Knowing which professionals are involved in a patient's care, how they work and their professional standing is key to working effectively within the healthcare team to ensure safe prescribing (Hammick et al., 2009). You therefore need to be able to define the different roles, responsibilities and expertise of a range of healthcare professionals in the prescribing process and MDT, as well as valuing all roles in terms of their contribution.

Time should be set aside for ensuring CPD and mentoring support, with provision made for MDTs to learn together.

One of the key barriers to MDT working relates to the culture of professions and the organisation. As a nurse prescriber you must be able to put the interests of patients before professional cultural norms and be prepared to work in different ways. For example, in the community these different ways of working include a focus on case management and support to provide home-based care rather than secondary care; joint care planning; co-ordinated assessments of care needs; named care co-ordinators who act as navigators and who retain responsibility for patient care and experiences throughout the patient journey; and clinical records that are shared across the MDT (NHS England, 2014; CordisBright, 2018). Effective MDTs develop over time and with experience. Collaborative cultures, trusting relationships and reflective team learning are at the heart of team working (NHS, 2021). Successful joint working requires clear, realistic and achievable aims and objectives, which are understood and accepted by all partners, including patients, families and carers. Key indicators of progress should be agreed, with buy in from all partners, recognising that there may be unintended consequences of introducing MDT working – for example, more preventative and personalised care may lead to a rise in unplanned hospital admissions (NHS, 2021), with possible duplication of tests and, in some cases, different practitioners repeating consultations. One of the key facilitators to working across boundaries is the optimal use of technology and allowing all members of the MDT 'real-time' access to patient records. This is linked with good communication, both verbal and electronic, as clear systems and protocols should be in place for how information about patients is shared not only within the MDT but also with other teams and, most importantly, with patients and carers (Baird et al., 2020).

As discussed in Chapter 5, we need to respect patients' beliefs and values; therefore, as well as working in partnership with colleagues for the benefit of patients you should endeavour to ascertain what the patient understands about their condition in addition to the source/s that led to such ideas and concerns. While their understanding may be underpinned by information gleaned through the internet, more often than not it is via a healthcare professional. Overtly dismissing these views increases the risk of breaking down your relationship with your patient. If you disagree with the views purported to originate from a particular professional, it is prudent to liaise with the relevant professional to seek clarification. Either way, the importance of working effectively with others, including partnership with your patients, with clear communication is paramount in optimising your patient's wellbeing. The development of specialist clinics such as musculoskeletal, ear, nose and throat, dermatology and adult hearing loss in GP practices rather than the hospital setting improves patient wellbeing by providing treatment by experienced specialist healthcare professionals, which may include advanced nurse practitioners, physiotherapists, pharmacists and physician associates as well as GPs. This brings care closer to where the patient lives, offers shorter waiting times and complete care in one visit.

As a nurse prescriber it is therefore key that you understand how the different practitioners work in your area of practice, and that you know each other's strengths and expertise and when to involve others for support. It is also important that your patients are made to feel involved with their treatment and understand why they may be seeing different healthcare professionals. Some patients, especially the elderly, may have been used to seeing only their GP and are now seeing a variety of practitioners, which can lead to confusion and misunderstanding. Communication with patients and carers and within the team is therefore key to avoiding any misunderstandings. A joint document published in 2020 by the RPS and the Royal College of General Practitioners entitled *Multidisciplinary Team Working in a Practice Setting* is a useful resource for you to read as it outlines the practicalities of making MDTs work. It covers communicating with patients and carers as well as communication within the MDT, stressing the need to ensure the frequency, timings and methods of how the team will communicate so it can function and make decisions effectively. It also has a useful section outlining the range of healthcare professionals who may be involved in your team with their possible roles and responsibilities (RPS, 2021). We conclude this chapter with a personal view from an advanced pharmacist practitioner who outlines their role in general practice and the enablers to working as part of an MDT.

Multidisciplinary teams in general practice: A personal view

As you know and have seen from the section above, MDTs have been part of the hospital secondary care structure of the NHS for many years. However, these are beginning to emerge in the general practice, primary care sector too. General practice has diversified in terms of staffing since the introduction of the Network Contract Directed Enhanced Service (DES) contract specification for primary care networks, as part of the aspiration to develop integrated care systems. You can see more on this development, including the full GP contract in *Primary Care Networks* (PCN, 2023).

How did general practice MDTs develop?

The development required practices to work in geographical groupings to improve patient care in their area and provided funding for a wide range of healthcare professionals not previously commonly encountered in general practice – for example, clinical pharmacists, physiotherapists, dietitians, advanced clinical practitioners, social prescribers and many more.

As a prescriber in general practice, you will be faced with a population with diverse needs ranging from those with single conditions to those with complex multimorbidity. Prescribing is increasingly complex, with many conditions managed principally in general practice, with advisory support from secondary or tertiary care. A wide multidisciplinary approach is essential, making use of the skills, knowledge and experience of the whole team who may have input into treating and supporting the patient.

Advanced pharmacist practitioners (APPs) working in general practice are independent prescribers that have trained in advanced clinical practice to be able to assess and diagnose within their competence.

Role of a specific advanced pharmacist practitioner in the MDT

The role is generally seeing people with diagnosed long-term conditions (LTC) for medicines optimisation, initiation, review, up-titration and sometimes deprescribing as a patient's status changes (e.g. increasing frailty).

I will sometimes help out with acute lists if the GPs are struggling, taking a history and then action on the issue if within my competence (which is growing over time in terms of clinical assessment and diagnosis, as it did with prescribing competency in more varied areas than my original specialism of neurology).

I am the prescribing lead for the practice (previously a GP role) which involves liaising with the ICB and keeping abreast of policy and guideline changes and medicines safety alerts etc., as well as ensuring these are briefed to the whole MDT. I lead on several clinical areas for the practice, including heart failure, shared care prescribing and cardiovascular disease. I am also increasingly the point of contact for the prescribing nurses when they need support – for example, with diabetes management. The other prescribing pharmacist at the practice takes a lead on mental health and medicines of potential misuse.

In the GP practice and PCN we are discussing here, there is a well-established MDT. As an APP based in one practice, I regularly discuss patients with nurses, GPs, advanced practitioners, social prescribers, mental health teams and secondary care clinicians, both to access support for my prescribing decisions in areas where I do not have in-depth knowledge and to provide support for others.

We run a variety of MDT meetings to bring appropriate staff members together to improve patient care. Each of our four care homes has a weekly virtual care home MDT via Microsoft Teams attended by GPs, a consultant geriatrician, clinical pharmacist, care home nurses, advanced nurse practitioners and care co-ordinators. This has greatly improved our relationships with the care homes and allowed the care homes' staff a forum in which to raise more routine matters that do not require an on-the-day GP visit, as well as allowing the practice a better overview of residents' health and care needs.

We also have a rotating series of weekly meetings at the practice covering palliative care, safeguarding, general clinical issues and prescribing updates. Again, these are run on an MDT footing, involving external stakeholders where appropriate – for example, hospice palliative care nurses or the children's home-visiting nurses – for the safeguarding meeting. At the palliative care meeting this has again improved whole-practice awareness of our palliative care patients and also allowed us to rapidly escalate patients for specialist input where needed.

We have recently taken part in a heart failure MDT pilot, where a weekly virtual clinical meeting is held via Teams. Practices can take cases to be discussed (with patient consent) and advice is provided by the consultant cardiologists. This may involve advice about next steps for prescribing, or rapid escalation of care to the community heart failure nurses or hospital heart failure consultants as needed.

Summary

Risk can be defined as a potential harmful outcome that can occur with a known or unknown probability. The risk of harm associated with medicine-taking typically refers to the likelihood of experiencing a side-effect associated with a treatment. All medicines can cause harm and the frequency and severity to which a person might experience a side-effect may vary from drug to drug.

One way to minimise risk is to work with colleagues and to know when you need support. Good practice is a thriving MDT with cross-speciality queries and advice and flows of information to better patient care. MDTs both in hospital and in general practice help support and potentially reduce risk associated with prescribing. Working collaboratively as part of that team can ensure a safe and effective transfer and continuity of care process is developed.

References

Akl, E.A., Oxman, A.D., Herrin, J., Vist, G.E., Terrenato, I., Sperati, F., Costiniuk, C., Blank, D. and Schünemann, H., 2011. Using alternative statistical formats for presenting risks and risk reductions. *Cochrane Database of Systematic Reviews*, (3).

Baird, B., Chauhan, K., Boyle, T., Heller, A. and Price, C. 2020. *How to Build Effective Teams in General Practice*. The King's Fund. Available at www.kingsfund.org.uk/publications/effective-teams-general-practice (accessed 30 March 2023).

Berry, D.C., Knapp, P.R. and Raynor, T., 2002. Is 15 per cent very common? Informing people about the risks of medication side effects. *International Journal of Pharmacy Practice*, 10(3), pp.145–151.

Berry, D.C., Raynor, D.K. and Knapp, P., 2003. Communicating risk of medication side effects: an empirical evaluation of EU recommended terminology. *Psychology, Health & Medicine*, 8(3), pp.251–263.

Berry, D. 2004. *Risk, Communication and Health Psychology*. Maidenhead: Open University Press.

Blalock, S.J., Dickinson, R. and Knapp, P. 2019. Risk evaluation and communication. In B. Strom, S. Kimmel and S. Hennessy (Eds.), *Pharmacoepidemiology*. 6th ed. Chichester: Wiley-Blackwell, pp. 1010–29.

Bogardus Jr, S.T., Holmboe, E. and Jekel, J.F., 1999. Perils, pitfalls, and possibilities in talking about medical risk. *Jama*, 281(11), pp.1037–1041.

Chan, S.W., Tulloch, E., Cooper, S.E., Smith, A. and Wojcik, W. 2017. Montgomery and informed consent: Where are we now? *British Medical Journal*. **357**, j2224.

CordisBright 2018. *What are the Key Factors for Successful Multidisciplinary Team Working?* Available at www.cordisbright.co.uk/admin/resources/05-hsc-evidence-reviews-multidisciplinary-team-working.pdf (accessed 30 March 2023).

Dickinson, R., Raynor, D., Knapp, P. and Macdonald, J. 2016. Providing additional information about the benefits of statins in a leaflet for patients with coronary heart disease: a qualitative study of the impact on attitudes and beliefs. *BMJ Open*, **6**, e012000.

Dickinson, R.J. 2014. The inclusion of a headline section and information about the benefits of medicines in written medicines information. PhD, University of Leeds.

Drug and Therapeutics Bulletin 2013. An introduction to patient decision aids. *British Medical Journal.* **347**, f4147.

Gigerenzer, G. 2011. What are natural frequencies? *British Medical Journal.* **343**, d6386.

Hammick, M., Freeth, D.S., Copperman, J. and Goodsman, D. 2009. *Being Interprofessional.* Fareham: CAIPE.

Hoffman, T.C. and Del Mar, C. 2015. Patients' expectations of the benefits and harms of treatments, screening, and tests: a systematic review. *JAMA Internal Medicine.* **175**, pp. 274–86.

Juanchich, M. and Sirota, M. 2020. Most family physicians report communicating the risks of adverse drug reactions in words (vs numbers). *Applied Cognitive Psychology.* **34**, pp. 526–34.

Knapp, P., Raynor, D.K., Silcock, J. and Parkinson, B., 2009. Performance-based readability testing of participant materials for a phase I trial: TGN1412. *Journal of Medical Ethics,* **35**(9), pp. 573–578.

MHRA 2005. *Always Read the Leaflet: Getting the Best Information with Every Medicine.* Medicines and Healthcare Products Agency. London: HMSO.

Mishel, M.H. 1990. Reconceptualization of the uncertainty in illness theory. *Image: The Journal of Nursing Scholarship.* **22**, pp. 256–62.

Montgomery v Lanarkshire Health Board 2015. S. [11]. AC 1430. Available at www.supremecourt.uk/cases/uksc-2013-0136.html (accessed April 2023).

NHS England 2014. *MDT Development: Working Toward an Effective Multidisciplinary/Multiagency Team.* Available at www.england.nhs.uk/wp-content/uploads/2015/01/mdt-dev-guid-flat-fin.pdf (accessed 30 March 2023).

NHS 2020. *We are the NHS: People Plan for 2020/21: Action for Us All.* Available at www.england.nhs.uk/ournhspeople/ (accessed 30 March 2023).

NHS 2021. *HEE Multidisciplinary Team (MDT): Toolkit.* Available at www.hee.nhs.uk/our-work/workforce-transformation/multidisciplinary-team-mdt-toolkit (accessed 30 March 2023).

NICE 2014. Cardiovascular disease: risk assessment and reduction, including lipid modification Clinical guideline [CG181].

NICE 2019. Bisphosphonates for treating osteoporosis Technology appraisal guidance [TA464].

NICE 2021. *Standards Framework for Shared Decision-making Support Tools, including Patient Decision Aids.* Available at www.nice.org.uk/corporate/ecd8 (accessed April 2023).

Oudhoff, J.P. and Timmermans, D.R. 2015. The effect of different graphical and numerical likelihood formats on perception of likelihood and choice. *Medical Decision Making.* **35**(4), pp. 487–500.

PCN 2023. *Primary Care Networks.* Available at www.england.nhs.uk/primary-care/primary-care-networks/network-contract-des/ (accessed 1 June 2023).

Politi, M.C., Han, P.K. and Col, N.F. 2007. Communicating the uncertainty of harms and benefits of medical interventions. *Medical Decision Making.* **27**, pp. 681–95.

Ranganathan, P., Pramesh, C. S., & Aggarwal, R. 2016. Common pitfalls in statistical analysis: Absolute risk reduction, relative risk reduction, and number needed to treat. *Perspectives in clinical research,* 7(1), 51.

RPS 2021. *A Competency Framework for All Prescribers.* Available at www.rpharms.com/resources/frameworks/prescribing-competency-framework/competency-framework (accessed 12 May 2023).

RPS and RCGP 2020. *Multidisciplinary Team Working in a General Practice Setting: The Practicalities of Making It Work.* Royal Pharmaceutical Society and Royal College of General Practitioners. Available at Multidisciplinary Team Working in a General Practice Setting (accessed 30 March 2023).

Stacey, D., Légaré, F., Lewis, K., Barry, M.J., Bennett, C.L., Eden, K.B., Holmes-Rovner, M., Llewellyn-Thomas, H., Lyddiatt, A., Thomson, R. and Trevena, L. 2017. Decision aids for people facing health treatment or screening decisions. *Cochrane Database of Systematic Reviews.* **4**(4), CD001431.

Stacey, D. and Volk, R.J. 2021. The International Patient Decision Aid Standards (IPDAS) Collaboration: Evidence update 2.0. *Medical Decision Making.* **41**(7), pp. 729–33.

Stone, E.R., Bruine de Bruin, W., Wilkins, A.M., Boker, E.M. and MacDonald Gibson, J. 2017. Designing graphs to communicate risks: Understanding how the choice of graphical format influences decision making. *Risk Analysis.* **37**(4), pp. 612–28.

Thorstensen-Woll, C., Wellings, D., Crump, H. and Graham, C. 2021. *Understanding Integration: How to Listen and Learn from People and Communities.* The King's Fund. Available at www.kingsfund.org.uk/publications/understanding-integration-listen-people-communities (accessed 30 March 2023).

Trevena, L.J, Bonner, C., Okan, Y., Peters, E., Gaissmaier, W., Han, P.K.J., Ozanne, E., Timmermans, D. and Zikmund-Fisher, B.J. 2021. Current challenges when using numbers in patient decision aids: Advanced concepts. *Medical Decision Making.* **41**(7), pp. 834–47.

Knapp, P., Raynor, D.K., Silcock, J. and Parkinson, B., 2009. Performance-based readability testing of participant materials for a phase I trial: TGN1412. *Journal of Medical Ethics,* 35(9), pp.573-578.

Van der Bles, A.M., Van der Linden, S. Freeman, A.L., Mitchell, J., Galvao, A.B., Zaval, L. and Spiegelhalter, D.J. 2019. Communicating uncertainty about facts, numbers and science. *Royal Society Open Science.* **6**(5), 181870.

5

Understanding Patients' Medicines-Related Values, Beliefs and Expectations and Safeguarding

Claire Easthall, Rebecca Dickinson, Ruth Setchell and Barry Strickland-Hodge

---

Chapter summary

This chapter supports prescribers to consider and respect patient diversity, values, beliefs and expectations about health and its treatment.

- It will address social and physical determinants of health, including general socioeconomic, cultural and environmental conditions and their influence on the patient and prescriber.
- It will include a discussion of religious requirements and preferences when offering specific medicines such as those of porcine or bovine derivative.
- It also explores safeguarding children and vulnerable adults, including possible signs of abuse, neglect, or exploitation, as well as focusing on both the patient's physical and mental health particularly if vulnerabilities may lead them to seek treatment unnecessarily or for the wrong reasons.

Introduction

The UK is home to a population with diversity of ethnicity, identity, language, religion, socio-economic status, sexual orientation, educational attainment, health, disability and caring commitments (Census, 2021). It is imperative that when making prescribing decisions nurses are self-aware enough to consider the influence of these key demographics on people's experiences of medicine-taking and how this may impact on people's preferences for treatment and treatment appropriateness. You have an ethical, moral and legal obligation to be self-aware regarding the provision of care that meets the needs of a diverse population in a way that promotes compassion, fairness, justice and equality and which does not discriminate.

Respecting patients' diversity

In the *Competency Framework for All Prescribers* (RPS, 2021a) Competency 3, Present options and reach a shared decision, has the supporting statement 3.2 'Considers and respects patient diversity, background, personal values and beliefs about their health, treatment and medicines, supporting the values of equality and inclusivity, and developing cultural competence'. In addition, Competency 2 is Identify evidence-based treatment options available. Supporting statement 2.6 is 'Considers any relevant patient factors and their potential impact on the choice and formulation of medicines, and the route of administration'. This is further explained as including an ability to swallow, disability, visual impairment, frailty, dexterity, religion, beliefs and intolerances.

Equality and diversity

Equality and diversity are core values associated with nursing practice. The NMC *Code* (NMC, 2018) underpins your practice and stipulates that you should provide person-centred care that promotes dignity and respect. These concepts should not be new to you; however, it is worth reflecting on these again in the context of how these might be considered in relation to prescribing practice.

Your actions as a nurse are guided by the law in this area. There are two main pieces of legislation that govern practice in relation to diversity, equality and inclusion. These are the Equality Act 2010 and the Human Rights Act 1998.

The Equality Act 2010

The Equality Act brought together several different pieces of legislation designed to end discrimination and promote equality. The Act stipulates that it is unlawful to discriminate against anyone based upon any of the protected characteristics shown in **Box 5.1**.

The Act identifies different ways in which people can be treated unfairly by defining manifestations of discrimination, harassment and victimisation. Discrimination may be direct, where it is overt that someone is being treated less favourably than others because of a protected characteristic. It might also be indirect, where someone with a protected characteristic is at a disadvantage because of rules or processes that result in unfavourable outcomes due to their protected characteristic.

Harassment occurs when a person is on the receiving end of unwanted behaviour that creates an offensive environment for them because of a protected characteristic. Victimisation is when someone is treated unfairly because they've complained about discrimination or harassment (Equality Act, 2010).

Box 5.1 Protected characteristics under the Equality Act 2010

Age
Disability
Gender reassignment
Marriage and civil partnership
Pregnancy and maternity
Race
Religion or belief
Sex
Sexual orientation

The Human Rights Act 1998

The Human Rights Act is a UK law passed in 1998. It lets you defend your rights in UK courts and compels public organisations – including the government, police and local councils – to treat everyone equally, with fairness, dignity and respect. It sets out the fundamental rights and freedoms that people in the UK can expect. The rights that UK citizens are entitled to are set out in a list of articles – for example, a right to life and freedom of expression. A key effect of the Act is that public bodies are expected to respect your rights; this applies to our healthcare and prescribing practice.

What does diversity in prescribing mean?

Diversity as related to prescribing means lots of different things, including the acknowledgement of different renal function, different metabolism and ethnic variations in responses to treatments and interventions (Harrison et al., 2020; Tamargo et al., 2017; Hudson-Sharpe and Metcalf, 2016). We mean diversity in terms of understanding patients as unique individuals with their own values, beliefs and expectations about health and medicines, which affect their treatment-related decisions and so, in turn, will affect your prescribing interactions with them.

Respecting and understanding patient diversity relates to understanding individual differences and accepting that not all of your patients are the same. In terms of prescribing an appropriate medicine, this could mean considering individual factors such as a patient's ethnicity – for example, it might affect the choice of which antihypertensive to prescribe (Eastwood et al., 2022; NICE, 2022b). Also see the section on religious beliefs later in this chapter.

We could also mean diversity in terms of differing comorbidities that affect our prescribing decisions – for example, the need to reduce the dose of a medicine prescribed to a patient with renal impairment (Wood et al., 2018; NICE, 2019). Issues such as these, relating to the individual variation in clinical factors that affect prescribing, are discussed in Chapter 8.

For this section, however, we are considering patient diversity in terms of the individual differences that occur through patients' values, beliefs and expectations about health and its treatment, specifically the prescribing of medicines.

Exploring patients' medicines-related values, beliefs and expectations

Understanding medicines use from the patient's perspective, to acknowledge their medicines-related values, beliefs, experiences and expectations, requires an open-minded, non-judgemental consultation style, where rapport and trust have been built. Active-listening and empathy are also key attributes. These consultation skills are not specific to exploring patients' medicines-related values, beliefs and expectations; they are considered in detail in Chapter 3 of this book.

Medicines optimisation: Understanding medicines use from the patients' perspective

As prescribers, we all need to ensure optimal use of medicines (NICE, 2015). This means ensuring treatment decisions are evidence-based and as safe as possible (see also Chapter 9, which considers drug interactions and adverse drug reactions). Optimising medicines use needs to be part of your routine practice as a prescriber and healthcare professional. However, it will not be optimal if the patients are not using the medicine as intended. The first principle of medicines optimisation, as defined by the RPS (2021b), is to aim to understand medicines use from the patients' perspective. This encompasses an ongoing and open dialogue with patients and/or their carers where patient choice is respected and their values, beliefs, expectations and experiences are acknowledged.

Worthy of note at this stage is consideration of what we actually mean by optimal medicines use, and recognition that person-centred care is at the heart of this. As healthcare professionals we sometimes forget just how much we ask of patients when we casually say, for example, take this antibiotic – four times a day on an empty stomach; we don't realise the potential added burden that it may be to follow the instructions that go with a medicine. In the case of the antibiotic, a full explanation of why this drug and why it needs to be spaced evenly through the day – ideally at six-hourly intervals – is important. An explanation that it is for short-term use might also help.

The correct definition of 'on an empty stomach' is shown in the recommended wording of the cautionary and advisory labels section of the BNF (number 23, which states to take the medicine one hour before or two hours after food). There are other occasions when 'before food' might mean 30 to 60 minutes before food and the number of the label is shown in the monograph of that medicine. For example, if you look up perindopril erbumine in the BNF, it gives the cautionary label 22 which states 'take 30 to 60 minutes before food'. These cautionary notes will be on the label of any dispensed medicine, but you can also see them in the BNF.

Medicines adherence

Medicines adherence describes the extent to which a patient's medicines use matches the agreed recommendations from the prescriber (Gast and Mathes, 2019; NICE, 2009). This broadly covers taking the correct quantity of the correct medicine, at the correct time, in the correct way. When we break this down further, we can see just how much needs to be in place to consider a patient as adherent to their medicines and, thus, the multitude of ways in which a patient may be non-adherent. We often think of medicines non-adherence as just the patient who does not take their medicines at all, or those who miss out doses, but it encapsulates any deviation from the intended way in which a medicine was planned to be used.

Competency 3 of the *Competency Framework* has the supporting statement 3.4: 'Assesses adherence in a non-judgemental way and understands the reasons for non-adherence and how best to support the patient/carer'. It represents a fundamental limitation in the delivery of healthcare, often because of a failure to fully agree the prescription in the first place or to identify and provide the support that patients need later on (NICE, 2009).

The World Health Organization (WHO) estimates that 30–50 per cent of medicines prescribed for long-term conditions are not taken as the prescriber intended, and subsequently describes medicines non-adherence as a worldwide problem of striking magnitude (NICE, 2015). As a prescriber, you need to understand the factors that may precipitate medicines non-adherence and we need to explore these at an individual level.

Medicine-taking is a complex health behaviour with an equally complex number of factors that influence this (Easthall, 2019). When we seek to resolve medicines non-adherence it is pertinent that this is through a person-centred and individualised approach; there is no one-size-fits-all approach to resolving medicines non-adherence. The resolution strategy needs to be tailored to meet individual need and bespoke to the adherence barriers experienced; we need to understand medicines use from the patient's perspective and respect their diversity.

You may have noted the terminology used here; 'medicines adherence' is a preferred term which implies some level of patient involvement and which is widely considered to be less judgemental than the term 'compliance', which implies a paternalistic, patriarchal relationship between the prescriber and patient (Horne et al., 2005; De las Cuevas, 2011). You'll likely hear the terms used interchangeably in practice and may indeed believe them to be synonymous yourself, but the subtleties in nomenclature here can make a real difference to the rapport-building stage of your patient consultation and thus your ability to understand medicines use from the patient's perspective.

Intentional and unintentional medicines non-adherence

Given medicine-taking is a complex health behaviour, it should come as no surprise to understand that the reasons patients do not take their medicines as prescribed are equally complex and multifaceted. There are a number of adherence determinants linked to both practical and perceptual barriers. A common way in which we define medicines non-adherence is to con-sider it as an intentional or unintentional act (Horne et al., 2005; Easthall and Barnett, 2017).

The National Institute for Health and Care Excellence (NICE) produced guidance in 2009 which covers most aspects of adherence including how to support the patient; which you are encouraged to look at.

Unintentional non-adherence describes patients who are willing to take their medicines as prescribed, but who cannot, usually due to some form of practical impediment such as cog-nitive deficits (e.g., memory loss) or dexterity issues (such as difficulty accessing medicines from their packaging). This is important not only for oral medicines but topical agents such as ointments. These often come in metal tubes and patients with, for example, rheumatoid arthritis or osteoarthritis may have significant difficulties getting the ointment out of the tube. Patients can, of course, talk to their local community pharmacist for support.

Unintentional non-adherence may also encompass difficulties such as visual impairment, lack of knowledge and understanding and swallowing difficulties, among others. Such non-adherence is determined by the patient's capability and opportunity to take their medicines as prescribed, rather than their motivation to do so. Interventions to resolve unintentional non-adherence should be focused on practical solutions to overcome the physical or cogni-tive deficits that impede adherence but should still be targeted to meet individual need.

Of course, it will not be possible to know what practical support is actually needed unless you have effectively used your consultation skills to understand medicines use from the patients' perspective and sought to understand the exact nature of the difficulties experi-enced. For patients who experience unintentional non-adherence, it is pertinent to recognise that these patients want to take their medicines but struggle to do so. Educating the patient on why they should and ought to take their medicine is unlikely to help (unless they genu-inely did not know what it was for or how they should be taking it) and in fact may lead a patient to feel disenfranchised and damage their trust in you. Similarly, trying to 'motivate' a patient to take their medicines when they are physically unable to do so may do more harm than good in terms of pushing the patient away and them not feeling understood.

The dosette box, or multi-compliance aid, is an intervention commonly provided to patients who may struggle to take their medicines due to issues with cognition or dexterity (Shenoy et al., 2020).

A person-centred assessment is required to understand if the provision of this interven-tion can help a person experiencing unintentional medication non-adherence; however, it is known that these will offer little benefit to those who have made a conscious decision not to take a medicine (intentional non-adherence) (Gast and Mathes, 2019; Bhattacharya et al., 2016). It is known that the use of compliance aids can increase some risks of harm associated with medicine-taking for some people (Bhattacharya et al., 2016) and, again, the importance of a person-centred exploration of the barriers to safe medicine-taking and the recommenda-tion of practical tailored solutions is essential.

Intentional non-adherence

Intentional non-adherence occurs when a patient makes a conscious decision not to take their medicines as prescribed, informed by factors such as their illness perceptions, health beliefs and emotions which in turn affect their motivation to adhere. These patients are able to take their medicines as prescribed but are unwilling to do so. An important observation here is recognition of the implicit judgement that may arise through describing a patient as unwilling to take their medicines as prescribed; there are subtle tones of wrong-doing implied, simply through the language used. As prescribers, you need to be mindful of this and ensure an open, non-judgemental exploration of patient preference and choice.

Interventions to support patients in resolving intentional non-adherence will tend to focus on increasing the patient's motivation to adhere, but this can only come through an in-depth exploration of the patient's perspectives and concerns. In terms of recognising individual diversity, it is essential to recognise patient choice and to be self-aware of our own perceptions too. For example, as a prescriber you might struggle to understand why a patient with severe eczema is refusing to use their emollient that we know will improve their condition; however, from the patient perspective, a lanolin-containing emollient (derived from sheep's wool) might be unacceptable to a vegan patient. Our own values and ideas may not match those of the patient and it is important that we are not quick to try and change an individual's perspective simply because it does not match our own.

A word of caution on differentiating between intentional and unintentional non-adherence. While considering non-adherence as intentional or unintentional can be helpful, such binary differentiations are not always reflective of reality; there are shades of grey in between. Consider, for example, a patient who states that they forget to take their medicine. We might assume this to be unintentional in nature, but actually, unless there are evidenced cognitive deficits, it could be that the patient forgets their medicine because they don't consider it as important, or perhaps there are competing priorities which come first. A behaviour that may superficially appear unintentional may actually have roots in illness perceptions and health beliefs, which fit more with the concept of intentional non-adherence, even if the patient is not aware of having made a conscious choice.

As prescribers, your role is to maintain an open-minded curiosity. Be mindful that when asked about medicines non-adherence, patients will often deflect to "I forget" as this is an easier answer to give than perhaps a more truthful response concerning fears, perceived social stigmas, emotions and so forth, that may precipitate an individual's choice to be non-adherent, but which may be difficult to disclose.

How can you help?

Apart from ensuring the patient is well informed about the medicine and how to take it, you may be able to help, particularly the unintentional non-adherent patient, by finding out what it is that is causing the issue. Is it timing or frequency of doses? If so, can you simplify the dosing regimen? An example might be diclofenac, which in its simple 50mg tablet form is taken three times a day, but offers a twice and once a day version which may help. If side-effects are the issue ensure you have discussed the potential for these at the consultation and describe how you could overcome them. It may be necessary to change the medicine completely. For example, if the patient complains of an irritating cough with an angiotensin converting enzyme (ACE) inhibitor for long-term treatment of hypertension which is stopping them taking it, would a Angiotensin type 2 receptor antagonist be a solution? Target your support and help to the patient's need. NICE suggests that patients record their medicine-taking (NICE, 2009).

If it is for a long-term condition this may be as difficult as taking the medicine in the first place. However, if it is for a short course of, say, antibiotics this might help.

Theoretical perspectives to help prescribers

This section will summarise a few theoretical perspectives. It will be useful to read more about these models and theories as they will be helpful to apply to the case study below to understand some of the reasons behind health and medicine-taking behaviours.

Social determinants of health – The Dahlgren-Whitehead rainbow

Dahlgren and Whitehead's (1991) model maps the relationship between the individual, their environment and disease. While it is not specifically tailored to medicine-taking it can be a useful framework to apply to health to understand how internal and external factors influence health inequalities that can predict behaviour. This model has been widely used by international and national organisations to develop a range of hypotheses about the determinants of health and their influence on health outcomes.

Health is influenced by multiple factors. Individual lifestyle factors, such as age, sex and genetics are placed at the centre of the model, but other influential external factors are also included as important determining factors of health. Social and community networks including communities, education, living and working conditions, housing and sanitation are identified as relevant and important determining factors for our health. These interact with broader socioeconomic, cultural and environmental factors.

Prescribers can use this model to explore and explain the complex processes which can determine people's health. Examples of the relevance of this model have already been covered throughout this book. For example, individual factors such as age and ethnicity might influence risk factors for disease and choice of treatment (see section above on diversity). People's socioeconomic status and access to outdoor space might influence the risk of prevalence of some diseases, such as COVID-19 (Mikolai et al., 2020). Cost of prescriptions can be a barrier to access to medicines. In the section on remote prescribing in Chapter 10, you can read about how access-suitable dependable technology and the internet can be a barrier to effective consultation and remote prescribing (Greenhalgh, 2021). These are just a few examples of how the social determinants of health might impact on health and medicine-taking. As a prescriber you should consider how these factors will impact your prescribing practice and upon the treatment options you recommend.

Health belief model

This model has been used for several decades to predict how individual beliefs about health might influence behaviour (Rosenstock, 1974). The model sets out six components that influence health outcomes and behaviours: perceived severity, perceived susceptibility, perceived benefits, perceived barriers, cues to action and self-efficacy. People's perceptions of these components combined with their ability to perform the recommended health behaviour will influence outcomes. Exploring people's perceptions about these components as part of a person-centred consultation might reveal influences that can be a barrier, or indeed facilitator, to optimal medicines use.

Beliefs about medicines: necessity–concerns framework

Horne's conceptual model sets out how underpinning beliefs about medicines can influence adherence (Horne and Weinman, 1999). The model explains how perceptions about the necessity for a medicine and concerns about the medicine interact in a multidimensional, relational way and can predict the likelihood that a patient will adhere to a treatment (Phillips et al., 2014). To simplify this model, it suggests that people are highly adherent to medicines perceived as highly necessary when few concerns are present and are more likely to be non-adherent to medicines perceived as high risk and unnecessary. There is evidence that the use of this model to explore perceptions on prescribed medicines can enhance the quality of prescribing decisions and improve adherence by better involving patients in shared decision-making (Horne et al., 2013).

The COM-B model

We have already seen how non-adherence is influenced by a patient's *capability and opportunity and motivation* to take their medicines as prescribed (see section above on intentional and unintentional adherence). A strength of the COM-B model (COM-B, 2023) is that it presents evidence-based theory in a way that is accessible to practitioners, allowing them to consider targeting of the support needed, according to the nature of issues affecting the person's behaviour. When supporting a patient who is not taking their medicines as prescribed, establishing whether it is their capability, opportunity or motivation to do so offers a real advantage in knowing how best to overcome the issues. A patient requiring practical support to overcome challenges with capability and opportunity needs very different advice compared to a patient requiring psychological support to overcome challenges with motivation (West and Michie, 2020).

In summary, there are many conceptual and psychological models that can be used to explain and explore medicine-taking behaviour. Knowledge of these is important because it can help prescribers undertake more detailed, extensive and patient-centred explorations of adherence and develop strategies that are tailored to individual needs and more likely to offer success for patients requiring support with medicine-taking.

Activity 5.1

Now spend some time reading around these models. You can apply the COM-B model to the scenarios below: try and identify the complex and interconnected factors that influence medicine-taking behaviour.

You have been introduced to several factors known to influence adherence to medicines, including the concepts of intentional and unintentional medicines adherence. It is important for prescribers to explore the difference between these concepts when working with patients to manage medicines – but do be aware that there are shades of grey between the two and it can be difficult to differentiate between the key issues. Some models associated with health and medicine-taking behaviour have also been presented as a method for you to explore some of the key challenges associated with this complex and challenging issue.

Medicines non-adherence is common, complex and relates to more than 'just missed doses' (Easthall, 2019). As a prescriber you need to prioritise the importance of understanding medicines use from the patient's perspective; to acknowledge their medicines-related values, beliefs, experiences and expectations requires an open-minded, non-judgemental consultation style, where rapport and trust have been built.

Case study 5.1

Richard Wilton is a 58-year-old builder who presents at A&E with an acute exacerbation of asthma which has previously been well controlled. He makes a good recovery following treatment with salbutamol nebulisers. As the prescribing nurse providing care for him you take the opportunity to discuss his asthma management with him, to help make sure this does not happen again.

He was brought into A&E by 'one of the lads' from the building site and you note that Richard appears to be particularly anxious about this. When Richard was initially too breathless to speak for himself, you asked this colleague about Richard's symptoms; he commented: 'I've never seen him use an inhaler; I didn't even know he had asthma.' The young colleague in question seems genuinely concerned, asking 'Will he be alright? He's really given us a scare as he's a top bloke; we always tease him a little saying he's a bit like our dad 'cos he's older, but he really is a great guy to have on site.'

Using your skills in patient-centred consultations, you make time to sit with Richard and find out what's been happening. After you have established a good rapport and gained his trust, he explains that he changed job six months ago and started working on a new site where all of his colleagues were many years younger than him; as he puts it 'I'm old enough to be their dad.' In his last role, where he worked with a group of colleagues of similar ages who he'd known for years, he used to use his inhaler as and when needed without too much bother – maybe two or three times a month on average when he felt a bit wheezy. Since changing his job, he's felt too embarrassed to use his inhaler on site in front of all the young lads as he's worried they'll think he's too slow and old and not up to the job. His asthma has gradually been getting worse over the last few months until today, when this has happened. You note that Richard seems to have a very good understanding of his condition and the need to use his salbutamol inhaler when needed, despite today's incident.

a. Would you consider Richard's non-adherence to be intentional in nature or unintentional? Explain your reasoning.
b. What do you think is the main driving factor behind his non-adherence? You could use the COM-B model to understand which aspects of the scenario may influence non-adherence.

Points for reflection

- This is a form of intentional non-adherence.
- The motivational aspect of the model, in particular automatic motivation – the emotional responses people experience in life, is particularly pertinent to this behaviour.
- You might want to explore the role of emotions, including perceptions of stigma, embarrassment and social norms.
- Approaches to support medicine-taking might include building confidence, understanding fears and working towards alleviating these fears and the use of a person-centred, non-judgemental consultation.

Considerations for prescribing in mental health conditions

Prescribing in mental health conditions carries its own set of considerations depending on the diagnosed illness, the person's insight into their illness and their beliefs about it, their capacity to make decisions and, uniquely, whether the patient is being treated under the Mental Health Act (1983). The range of mental health conditions is large, including schizophrenia, bipolar disorder, dementia, depression, anxiety, attention deficit hyperactivity disorder, personality disorder and addiction. Gender services also currently fall within mental health service provision. The needs and vulnerabilities of these populations are extremely varied. As a prescriber you should have specialist expertise not only in the condition for which you prescribe, but also the age of the population and the setting. Treatment considerations within a psychiatric intensive care unit are very different to that in a mental health team in the community and are different again in primary care.

The *Competency Framework for All Prescribers* (RPS, 2021a) touches on mental health and safeguarding – for example, in Competency 1, Assess the patient, statement 1.8, it identifies and addresses potential vulnerabilities that may be causing the patient or carer to seek treatment. This is explained in the further information section as focusing on both the patient's physical and mental health, particularly if vulnerabilities may lead them to seek treatment unnecessarily or for the wrong reasons.

The social stigma surrounding mental health and its treatment is changing as it is being addressed in the media and public health campaigns (Henderson et al., 2020). Illness, diagnosis and treatment can, however, have a profound effect on a person's life and employment, and this may cause a person to initially avoid diagnosis or contact with mental health services and reject potentially beneficial treatment. For example, a person with prolonged low mood, poor sleep and lack of enjoyment of activities, feeling that life is not worth living (potentially with a moderate depression), may have a family member telling them they can 'sort themselves out' by going to the gym. They may also be worried about their employment if they are diagnosed with depression, have concerns about antidepressants being addictive and that they will be taking them for the rest of their lives. Whereas clinical trials show that antidepressants are an effective treatment for moderate to severe depression (Cipriani et al., 2018) and reduce the risk of death by suicide (Henriksson and Isacsson, 2006). For a first episode they can be stopped six months to a year after response (Reimherr et al., 1998), which can be assessed clinically and on validated depression rating scales appropriate to the setting (Willacy, 2019). Some antidepressants need dose tapering to prevent discontinuation effects, but they are not addictive. Additionally, NICE guidance states that adults diagnosed with moderate depression should be offered various treatment options including medication, psychotherapy and structured exercise (NICE, 2022a). Exercise has been shown to improve symptoms of mild and moderate depression, but there is less evidence for effect and relapse prevention than for psychological therapies and medication. People with moderate depression may benefit from regular contact with health professionals (Cooney et al., 2013).

By contrast, a patient with severe anxiety may have a short course of benzodiazepines prescribed. This may work well in helping them to relax and sleep and this person may put considerable pressure on you as a prescriber to repeat a prescription despite continuing courses of benzodiazepines causing addiction, reducing cognition and increasing falls (NICE, 2011).

A person with bipolar disorder could have multiple episodes of hypomania where their insight into their illness and capacity to make decisions fluctuates. Sometimes they will write an 'advanced decision' when they have capacity to make decisions to advise medical and social care staff of their wishes in times when they lack capacity (Mental Capacity Act, 2005; Mind, 2017). As a prescriber you need to be aware of such directives and be aware of their implications for prescribing. An advanced directive may include an agreement to be prescribed antipsychotic medication in an episode of hypomania in anticipation of them refusing it. Including families in the support of many patients is helpful but communication with them may be precluded by the advanced decision.

If you intend to prescribe for a person who lacks capacity to make decisions regarding treatment, their best interests must be taken into account (NICE, 2018; NICE, 2020); among other things, their views and beliefs when they did have capacity have to be considered. This can be difficult for families and carers when past choices have been felt to be unwise. For example, a person who is prescribed medication for high blood pressure consistently chooses not to take tablets despite knowing the stroke risk associated and the entreaties of their family. They subsequently have a stroke and develop vascular dementia. Their function deteriorates, requiring medication administering via a nasogastric tube and now lack capacity to make decisions regarding treatment. This person becomes very agitated at times when medication is administered so that most doses are missed. The person's earlier decision to refuse prophylactic medication should be taken into consideration in a multidisciplinary best interest meeting regarding the continuation of medication (BMA, 2019).

Practical issues encountered with medicines and religious beliefs

As a prescriber, you must consider the patient's beliefs – religious, cultural or other – and involve them in all aspects of the prescribing consultation.

Before initiating the consultation, always review the patient's current medical notes as any issues relating to the use of animal-derived medicines may have already been documented or raised with you. If there is no entry, remember to update the records with the details of your discussion as appropriate. There are a number of religious groups who will not accept substances taken from animals, in particular pigs or cows. Patients are much more likely to adhere to your suggested medicine recommendations if they are actively involved in the decision-making process and their beliefs are constructively considered.

In the *Competency Framework for All Prescribers* (RPS, 2021a) Competency 2, Identify evidence-based treatment options available for clinical decision-making, has the supporting statement: 2.6 'Considers any relevant patient factors and their potential impact on the choice and formulation of medicines, and the route of administration'.

In addition, Competency 3, Present options and reach a shared decision, has the supporting statement: 3.2 'Considers and respects patient diversity, background, personal values and beliefs about their health, treatment and medicines, supporting the values of equality and inclusivity, and developing cultural competence'; further information says: b 'In line with legislation requirements which apply to equality, diversity and inclusion'. Supporting statement 3.1 requires the prescriber to work in partnership with the patient to make informed choices, agreeing a plan that respects the patient's preference including their right to refuse or limit treatment. Other parts of Competency 3 are also valid at this point.

Are you aware of your patient's religious beliefs or preferences? Effective communication is essential for your role as a prescriber and you need to develop a good general knowledge of issues relating to prescribing for different religious groups. Knowledge of your patient's religious beliefs is important for you as a prescriber. Informed consent must be obtained from all patients by all prescribers. Questions to ask yourself include: have you made the patient aware that their treatment may include medicines derived from animals? If you have not, why is this?

This short section provides guidance as to how to respond to and assist patients wishing to avoid animal products, helping them to make informed decisions about their treatment. You may not have thought about his aspect of prescribing but it is important and there are useful texts to guide you. One from the government of Queensland, Australia, is particularly helpful. It is called *Medicines/pharmaceuticals of Animal Origin*; it was updated in 2020 (Queensland Health, 2020). We expect our prescribing practice to be patient-centred as this can improve the patient's experience and their adherence to the choice of medicines made. Many medicines and many different dosage forms contain or are derived from animal products. This includes tablets, capsules, creams, ointments and vaccines. Gelatin is usually derived from bovine or porcine collagen. Gelatin is used in making capsule shells, for example, but is also used as a stabiliser added to other pharmaceutical products such as vaccines. Faiths such as Muslim, Christian, Jewish, Hindu and Buddhist have specific restrictions for the use of animal products. Other individual groups may have ethical reasons for not wishing to use animal-derived products, which will include the use of medicines and vaccines. Not all members of a particular group will necessarily have the same view on this. The issue really arises when you are wishing to recommend a medicine which is known to be of animal derivation and where there is no synthetic alternative available. Although medicines derived from pigs could potentially be an issue for many faiths it is more likely to be an issue for people of Judaism and Islamic faiths.

This is relevant when substances have been converted into something else with different characteristics, thus changing the substance potentially into a pure form from an impure form for those from particular religious groups. According to a paper by WHO (2001): 'The gelatin formed as a result of the transformation of the bones, skin and tendons of a judicially impure animal is pure and it is judicially permissible to eat it.'

It is worth noting that necessities overrule prohibitions. For Jewish patients, any food or dietary additive or medicine that is to be swallowed must contain only kosher ingredients.

There has been a move from biologically sourced to synthetic forms of drugs. However, the animal origin of any drug treatment should form part of all clinical decision-making. Low molecular weight heparins, for example, may be porcine-derived, but there is a synthetic preparation available – fondaparinux. Patients who have specific requirements or preferences should be offered a choice if a choice exists and, if it does not, then this needs to form part of the consultation. For information as to whether a medicine is of animal origin, use the online resource www.medicines.org.uk to view the Summary of Product Characteristics (SmPC), or contact the manufacturer directly. Not all medicines are covered but the majority are.

As prescribers, knowledge of a patient's preferences in relation to animal-derived medications inform the decision-making process when selecting a medication. This, ultimately, may help to ensure adherence by patients and reduce costs associated with non-adherence.

Although the above brief discussion was looking at religion you may well be asked about drugs of animal origin for vegetarians or vegans. For example, as the UK-based Vegan Society observes, 'we live in an imperfect world'. In the Vegan Society's Memorandum of Association, veganism is used to denote a philosophy and way of living which seeks to exclude – as far as possible and practicable – all forms of exploitation of, and cruelty to, animals. 'You yourself know best what your own particular situation is, what efforts you can make and what possible and practicable means for you' In the Queensland Health document of 2020, two blogs are identified. The Vegan Society (England and Wales) has two blogs about medication (2017 a and b). Queensland Health (2020) also lists a number of faiths with their dietary restrictions.

Safeguarding: The role of the prescriber

Safeguarding is everybody's business (gov.uk, 2019). To provide high-quality, safe and effective care to patients you need to be able to apply the principles and duties of safeguarding to people requiring pharmaceutical care.

In the *Competency Framework for All Prescribers* (RPS, 2021a), Competency 1 is Assess the patient and supporting statement 1.8 states: 'Identifies and addresses potential vulnerabilities that may be causing the patient/carer to seek treatment'. In the further information section, it says: g 'Safeguarding children and vulnerable adults (possible signs of abuse, neglect, or exploitation), and focusing on both the patient's physical and mental health, particularly if vulnerabilities may lead them to seek treatment unnecessarily or for the wrong reasons'. In Competency 4, Prescribe, support statement 4.7 states: 'Recognises potential misuse of medicines; minimises risk and manages using appropriate processes'. Further information also states: d 'Minimises risk by ensuring appropriate safeguards are in place''

As a nurse, you will already have a professional, legal and moral obligation to protect vulnerable adults and children from harm and perform safeguarding duties (NMC, 2018). You should already be aware of the six principles of safeguarding that are embedded in the Care Act (2014); these apply to all health and care settings (see Box 5.2). This section sets out the principles of safeguarding and considers these in relation to prescribing practice.

Safeguarding is defined in the Care Act (2014) as follows:

> Protecting an adult's right to live in safety, free from abuse and neglect. It is about people and organisations working together to prevent and stop both the risks and experience of abuse or neglect, while at the same time making sure that the adult's wellbeing is promoted including, where appropriate, having regard to their views, wishes, feelings and beliefs in deciding on any action. This must recognise that adults sometimes have complex interpersonal relationships and may be ambivalent, unclear or unrealistic about their personal circumstances.

All people are potentially at risk of abuse, although there are populations who are more vulnerable to such risks (NHS England, 2022). Children and those who lack capacity, for example, are at increased risk of abuse and may require additional consideration. It is important to point out at this point that the principles of the Mental Capacity Act (2005) set out the assumption that adults have capacity to make decisions about themselves, so do keep this in mind.

You should already be aware of how to safeguard and have knowledge about some key concepts relating to safeguarding, such as the potential for abuse and neglect. Abuse can take many forms and may include any combination of the following: physical abuse, domestic violence or abuse, sexual abuse, psychological or emotional abuse, financial or material abuse, modern slavery, discriminatory abuse, organisational or institutional abuse, neglect or acts of omission and self-neglect (DHSC, 2023). Medication-related incidents can constitute a safeguarding issue and may well take one or more of the forms mentioned above. Medication-related incidents may arise due to poor practice, neglect, misuse of drugs and involve the use of medications intended to cause restriction or harm, an example being the use of antipsychotics as a so-called 'chemical cosh' for people with dementia. You have a duty of care to be observant for the presence of medication-related incidents and to act in a way that promotes the safe and effective use of medicines. You also have a duty of candour to escalate concerns if you have any (NMC, 2018). It is important to stay vigilant and observant for issues with the medications that might indicate a breach in safeguarding. This means that you, as a nurse, must tell the person (or, where appropriate, their advocate, carer or family) when something has gone wrong, apologise and offer an appropriate remedy or support to put matters right (if possible).

If you are concerned about a medicine-related safeguarding issue then it is essential that you raise your concerns straight away. You can speak to your manager or safeguarding lead. If you are concerned that a crime has been committed then report to the police. Familiarise yourself with your organisation's safeguarding policies, including the whistle-blowing policy, and remember that safeguarding is everybody's business.

Box 5.2 Six principles of safeguarding

Empowerment

People being supported and encouraged to make their own decisions and give informed consent.

Prevention

It's better to take action before mistreatment occurs.

Proportionality

The least intrusive response necessary to the risk presented.

Protection

Support and representation for those in greatest need.

Partnership

Working in partnership to achieve local solutions in communities where we live. Communities have a part to play in preventing, detecting and reporting abuse and neglect.

Accountability

Accountability and transparency in delivering safeguarding and fulfilling our duty of candour.

Case studies: safeguarding

Case study 5.2

Craig Jenkins is 75 years old; he has a diagnosis of vascular dementia. Craig can currently support his own care needs but cannot live independently because he can easily become confused. He lives with his nephew, Marcus, and his family in an annex at Marcus's property. Craig requires support from his family to prompt him to complete his activities of daily living and he needs support to manage his medicines because, although he knows what his medicines are for, he can become confused with which one is which. Marcus has previously reported that Craig is becoming more restless at night, which has caused some disruption to the family routine and resulted in Craig being more tired in the morning.

Craig visits you as the nurse prescriber after a fall at home. He says he has been feeling particularly drowsy in the morning recently and that this contributed to his fall.

You identify that there has recently been an increase in requests for a prescription for Chlorphenamine 4mg, which Craig has used for a long time to manage occasional bouts of urticaria.

- Are there any potential safeguarding concerns with this scenario?
- Is there a potential risk of harm in this scenario?
- Can you identify the safeguarding policies in your clinical area for escalating concerns?

Points for reflection

There is a possibility that the medication is being given as a form of restraint to prevent night-time wanderings. It might be possible that the family are not coping with the current situation and that a safeguarding concern needs to be generated. There is a risk of harm from falls related to the side-effects from the medication. Please identify the appropriate safeguarding policy in your field of practice.

Case study 5.3

You are visiting a patient in a care home to review a prescription, when visiting you observe a medication round in process. A patient is very distressed about being offered a medication. The patient shouts loudly and angrily that the nurse is trying to poison them and refuses the medication. The nurse leaves with the medication and a little while later returns with a chocolate mousse. You observe the nurse breaking the capsule, pouring the contents into the chocolate mousse and feeding this to the patient. In the patient's care records you cannot identify a specific plan that stipulates this is an acceptable action.

- Are there any potential safeguarding concerns with this scenario?
- Is there a potential risk of harm in this scenario?
- Can you identify the safeguarding policies in your clinical area for escalating concerns?

Points for reflection

The medication has been administered covertly without due process and this is a safeguarding concern. This will need to be escalated and reported. There is a risk of harm as there is potential for incorrect dosages because of changes to the properties of the medication. There is an issue with lack of informed consent from the patient. This action might constitute a type of neglect and act of omission for the following reasons.

- It could provide care in a way that the person dislikes.
- There is a failure to administer medication as prescribed.
- It is potentially preventing a person from making their own decisions.
- There is a failure to ensure privacy and dignity in care provision.

Summary

The chapter reminded prescribers to consider and respect patient diversity, values, beliefs and expectations about their health and treatment. It discussed the two main pieces of legislation that govern practice in relation to diversity, equality and inclusion. These are the Equality Act 2010 and the Human Rights Act 1998. It included the social and physical determinants of health and their influence on the patient and prescriber. The chapter considered religious requirements and preferences when offering specific medicines such as those of porcine or bovine derivative. Finally, it explored safeguarding children and vulnerable adults.

References

Badreldin, N., Grobman, W.A. and Yee, L.M. 2019. Racial disparities in postpartum pain management. *Obstetrics and Gynecology.* **134**(6), pp. 1147–53.

Bhattacharya, D., Aldus, C.F., Barton, G., Bond, C.M., Boonyaprapa, S., Charles, I.S., Fleetcroft, R., Holland, R., Jerosch-Herold, C., Salter, C., Shepstone, L., Walton, C., Watson, S. and Wright, D.J. 2016. The feasibility of determining the effectiveness and cost-effectiveness of medication organisation devices compared with usual care for older people in a community setting: Systematic review, stakeholder focus groups and feasibility randomised controlled trial. *Health Technology Assessment.* **20**(50).

BMA 2019. *Best Interest Decision Making for Adults Who Lack Capacity: A Toolkit for Doctors Working in England and Wales.* Available at www.bma.org.uk/media/1850/bma-best-interests-toolkit-2019.pdf (accessed 23 November 2022).

Care Act 2014. Available at www.legislation.gov.uk/ukpga/2014/23/contents/enacted (accessed 1 June 2023).

Census 2021. Available at census.gov.uk/census-2021-results (accessed 13 September 2023).

Cipriani, A., Furukawa, T.A., Salanti, G., Chaimani, A., Atkinson, L.Z., Ogawa, Y., Leucht, S., Ruhe, H.G., Turner, E.H., Higgins, J.P.T., Egger, M., Takeshima, N., Hayasaka, Y., Imai, H., Shinohara, K., Tajika, A., Ioannidis, J.P.A. and Geddes, J.R. 2018. Comparative efficacy and acceptability of 21 antidepressant drugs for the acute treatment of adults with major depressive disorder: a systematic review and network meta-analysis. *The Lancet.* **391**(10128), pp. 1357–66.

COM-B 2023. *The COM-B Model for Behavior Change.* The Decision Lab. Available at thedecisionlab.com/reference-guide/organizational-behavior/the-com-b-model-for-behavior-change (accessed June 2023).

Cooney, G., Dwan, K., Greig, C.A., Lawlor, D.A., Rimer, J., Waugh, F.R., McMurdo, M. and Mead, G.E. 2013. *Exercise for Depression.* Cochrane database of Systematic Reviews. 9 Art no CD004366.

Dahlgren, G., Whitehead, M. 1991. Policies and Strategies to Promote Social Equity in Health. Stockholm, Sweden: Institute for Futures Studies.

De las Cuevas, C. 2011. Towards a clarification of terminology in medicine taking behavior: Compliance, adherence and concordance are related although different terms with different uses. *Current Clinical Pharmacology.* **6**(2), pp. 74–7.

Department of Health and Social Care (DHSC) 2023. *Care And Support Statutory Guidance.* Available at www.gov.uk/government/publications/care-act-statutory-guidance/care-and-support-statutory-guidance (accessed 12 February 2023).

Easthall, C. 2019. Medication nonadherence as a complex health behavior: There is more to it than just missed doses. *Journal of the American Geriatric Society.* **67**, pp. 2439–40.

Easthall, C. and Barnett, N. 2017. Using theory to explore the determinants of medication adherence: Moving away from a one-size-fits-all approach. *Pharmacy.* **5**(3), p. 50.

Eastwood, S.V., Hughes, A.D., Tomlinson, L., Mathur, R., Smeeth, L., Bhaskaran, K. and Chaturvedi, N. 2022. Ethnic differences in hypertension management, medication use and blood pressure control in UK primary care, 2006–2019: A retrospective cohort study. *Lancet Regional Health Europe.* **25**, p. 100557.

Gast, A. and Mathes, T. 2019. Medication adherence influencing factors: An (updated) overview of systematic reviews. *Systems Revue.* **8**, p. 112

Göran, D. and Whitehead, M., 1991. Policies and strategies to promote social equity in health.

Greenhalgh, T., Rosen, R., Shaw, S.E., Byng, R., Faulkner, S., Finlay, T., Grundy, E., Husain, L., Hughes, G., Leone, C. and Moore, L., 2021. Planning and evaluating remote consultation services: a new conceptual framework incorporating complexity and practical ethics. *Frontiers in Digital Health*, 3, p.726095.

Gov.uk 2019. *Safeguarding Strategy 2019 to 2025: Office of the Public Guardian.* Available at www.gov.uk/government/publications/safeguarding-strategy-2019-to-2025-office-of-the-public-guardian/safeguarding-strategy-2019-to-2025-office-of-the-public-guardian (accessed 113 September 2023).

Harrison, E.M., Docherty, A.B., Barr, B., Buchan, I., Carson, G., Drake, T.M., Dunning, J., Fairfield, C.J., Gamble, C., Green, C.A., Griffiths, C., Halpin, S., Hardwick, H.E., Ho, A., Holden, K.A., Hollinghurst, J., Horby, P.W., Jackson, C., Katikireddi, S.V. et al. 2020. *Ethnicity and Outcomes from COVID-19: The ISARIC CCP-UK Prospective Observational Cohort Study of Hospitalised Patients.* Available at ssrn.com/abstract=3618215 or dx.doi.org/10.2139/ssrn.3618215 (accessed 13 September 2023).

Henderson, C., Potts, L. and Robinson, E. 2020. Mental illness stigma after a decade of Time to Change England: Inequalities as targets for further improvement. *European Journal of Public Health.* **30**(3), pp. 497–503.

Henriksson, S. and Isacsson, G. 2006. Increased antidepressant use and fewer suicides in Jämtland county, Sweden, after a primary care educational programme on the treatment of depression. *Acta Psychiatrica Scandinavica.* **114**, pp. 159–67.

Horne, R. and Weinman, J. 1999. Patients' beliefs about prescribed medicines and their role in adherence to treatment in chronic physical illness. *Journal of Psychosomatic Research.* **47**(6), pp. 555–67.

Horne, R, Chapman, S.C.E., Parham, R., Freemantle, N., Forbes, A. and Cooper, V. 2013. Understanding patients' adherence-related beliefs about medicines prescribed for long-term conditions: A meta-analytic review of the necessity–concerns framework. *PLoS One.* **8**(12).

Horne, R., Weinman, J., Barber, N., Elliott, R. and Morgan, M. 2005. *Concordance, Adherence and Compliance in Medicine Taking.* London: NCCSDO. **40**, p. 6.

Hudson-Sharpe, N. and Metcalf, H. 2016. *Inequality Among Lesbian, Gay Bisexual and Transgender Groups in the UK: A Review of Evidence.* London: National Institute of Economic and Social Research.

Mental Health Act 1983. UK Public General Acts. 1983. Mental Health Act (revised). Available at www.legislation.gov.uk/ukpga/1983/20/contents (accessed 16 November 2022).

Mental Capacity Act 2005. UK Public General Acts. Mental Capacity Act (revised) sections 24, 25 and 26. Available at www.legislation.gov.uk/ukpga/2005/9/part/1/crossheading/advance-decisions-to-refuse-treatment (accessed 27 November 2022).

Mikolai, J., Keenan, K. and Kulu, H. 2020. Intersecting household-level health and socio-economic vulnerabilities and the COVID-19 crisis: An analysis from the UK. *SSM – Population Health.* **12**, 100628.

Mind. 2017. Mental Capacity Act 2005 Advanced Decisions. Available at www.mind.org.uk/information-support/legal-rights/mental-capacity-act-2005/advance-decisions/ (accessed 27 November 2022).

NHS England 2022. *Safeguarding Children, Young People and Adults at Risk in the NHS.* Safeguarding accountability and assurance framework. Available at www.england.nhs.uk/wp-content/uploads/2015/07/B0818_Safeguarding-children-young-people-and-adults-at-risk-in-the-NHS-Safeguarding-accountability-and-assuran.pdf (accessed 25 October 2022).

NICE 2009. *Medicines Adherence: Involving Patients in Decisions About Prescribed Medicines and Supporting Adherence: Clinical Guideline [CG76]* Available at www.nice.org.uk/guidance/cg76 (accessed April 2023).

NICE 2011. *Generalised Anxiety Disorder and Panic Disorder in Adults: Management. (Updated 2020): Clinical Guideline CG113.* Available at www.nice.org.uk/guidance/cg113 (accessed 16 November 2022).

NICE 2018. *Decision-making and Mental Capacity: Clinical Guideline NG108.* Available at www.nice.org.uk/guidance/ng108 (accessed 22 November 2022).

NICE 2019. *Acute Kidney Injury: Prevention, Detection and Management [NG148].* London: NICE.

NICE 2020. *Decision-making and Mental Capacity: Quality Standard [QS194]. Best Interest Decision Making: Quality Statement 4.* Available at www.nice.org.uk/guidance/qs194/chapter/quality-statement-4-best-interests-decision-making (accessed 22 November 2022).

NICE 2022a. *Depression in Adults. Treatment and Management: Guideline NG222.* Available at www.nice.org.uk/guidance/ng222 (accessed 27 November 2022).

NICE 2022b. *Hypertension in Adults: Diagnosis and Management [NG136].* London: NICE.

NMC 2018. *The Code: Professional Standards of Practice and Behaviour for Nurses, Midwives and Nursing Associates.* Available at www.nmc.org.uk/globalassets/sitedocuments/nmc-publications/nmc-code.pdf (accessed 1 June 2023).

Phillips, L.A., Diefenbach, M., Kronish, I.M., Negron, R.M. and Horowitz, C.R. 2014. The necessity–concerns framework: A multidimensional theory benefits from multidimensional analysis. *Annals of Behavioral Medicine.* **48**(1), pp. 7–16.

Queensland Health 2020. *Medicines/pharmaceuticals of Animal Origin.* Available at www.health.qld.gov.au/__data/assets/pdf_file/0024/147507/qh-gdl-954.pdf (accessed 13 September 2023).

Reimherr, F.W., Amsterdam, J.D., Quitkin, F.M., Rosenbaum, A.F., Fava, M., Zajecka, J., Beasley Jr, C.M., Michelson, D., Roback, P. and Sundell, K. 1998. Optimal length of continuation therapy in depression: A prospective assessment during long-term fluoxetine treatment. *American Journal of Psychiatry.* **155**(9), pp. 1247–53.

Rosenstock, I.M. 1974. Historical origins of the health belief model. *Health Education Monographs.* **2**(4), pp. 328–35.

RPS 2021a. *A Competency Framework for All Prescribers.* Available at www.rpharms.com/resources/frameworks/prescribing-competency-framework/competency-framework (accessed 12 May 2023).

RPS 2021b. *Medicines Optimisation: How Patients Use Medicines Over Time.* Available at www.rpharms.com/resources/pharmacy-guides/medicines-optimisation (accessed 1 June 2023).

Shenoy, R., Scott, S. and Bhattacharya, D. 2020. Quantifying and characterising multi-compartment compliance aid provision. *Research in Social and Administrative Pharmacy.* **16**(4), pp. 560–7.

Tamargo, J., Rosano, G., Walther, T., Duarte, J., Niessner, A., Kaski, J.C., Ceconi, C., Drexel, H., Kjeldsen, K., Savarese, G., Torp-Pedersen, C., Atar, D., Lewis, B.S., and Agewall, S. 2017. Gender differences in the effects of cardiovascular drugs. *European Heart Journal: Cardiovascular Pharmacotherapy.* **3**(3), pp.163–82.

Vegan Society 2017a. *Is My Medication Vegan?* Available at www.vegansociety.com/news/blog/my-medication-vegan (accessed December 2022).

Vegan Society 2017b. *What Vegans Should Know Pre-operatively.* Available at: www.vegansociety.com/whats-new/blog/what-vegans-should-know-pre-operatively (accessed December 2022).

West, R. and Michie, S. 2020. A brief introduction to the COM-B model of behaviour and the PRIME theory of motivation (v1). *Qeios. Open access.* Article WW04E6.

While, A. 2020. Medication adherence: Understanding the issues and finding solutions. *British Journal of Community Nursing.* **2**(11), pp. 474–9.

WHO 2001. *Judicially Prohibited and Impure Substances in Foodstuff and Drugs.* Available at www.immunize.org/talking-about-vaccines/porcine.pdf (accessed 13 September 2023).

Willacy, H. 2019. *Screening for Depression in Primary Care: Patient, Professional Articles/Mental Health (Psychiatry).* Available at patient.info/doctor/screening-for-depression-in-primary-care (accessed 16 November 2022).

Willmott, T.J., Pang, B. and Rundle-Thiele, S. 2021. Capability, opportunity, and motivation: An across contexts empirical examination of the COM-B model. *BMC Public Health.* **21**, 1014.

Wood, S., Petty, D., Glidewell, L. and Raynor, D.T. 2018. Application of prescribing recommendations in older people with reduced kidney function: A cross-sectional study in general practice. *British Journal of General Practice.* **68**(670).

6

An Introduction to Pharmacology and Therapeutics and Prescribing Antimicrobials

Barry Strickland-Hodge, Joe Spencer-Jones and Rebecca Dickinson

Chapter summary

There are many textbooks which explain and discuss pharmacology and therapeutics. They are regularly updated and should be used if you would like to go into this subject in more detail. There are those which recommend pharmacology for nurses, but we think it is best, if you can and if you have the opportunity, to look at a few of these textbooks and decide which you prefer. A few are listed at the end of this section of the chapter.

This chapter considers:

* pharmacokinetics
* pharmacodynamics
* pharmacogenetics and pharmacogenomics.

It ends with a detailed section on antimicrobial prescribing, which sets out the concepts of antimicrobial resistance and antimicrobial stewardship and offers a practical exploration of principles of safe prescribing of antimicrobials, including reference to important principles of infection prevention and control.

It discusses the need for particular care when considering prescribing antimicrobials and infection prevention control. This includes antimicrobial stewardship. Antibiotic resistance and local policies to help prevent this will be discussed.

Introduction

In the *Competency Framework for All Prescribers* (RPS, 2021), Competency 2 is entitled Identify evidence-based treatment options available for clinical decision-making; there are a number of supporting statements, as well as further information, that relate to the subject of pharmacology – for example, supporting statement 2.1: 'Considers both non-pharmacological and pharmacological treatment approaches' and 2.2: 'Considers all pharmacological treatment options including optimising doses as well as stopping treatment (appropriate polypharmacy and deprescribing)'. Some of these topics have been or will be covered in other chapters. This one concentrates on pharmacokinetics, pharmacodynamics and briefly introduces pharmacogenomics and pharmacogenetics. In the further information of the *Competency Framework* (RPS, 2021) there is the statement that you as the prescriber should apply an understanding of the pharmacokinetics and pharmacodynamics of medicines, and how these may be altered by individual patient factors where these include genetics, age, renal impairment and pregnancy. Care with prescribing in specific patient groups such as these is covered in Chapter 8.

Pharmacology: What is it?

Pharmacology is not a single-strand science; it is the way the body acts on medicines, which is pharmacokinetics, and how the medicine acts on the body to have its effect, which is pharmacodynamics. Two newer areas to consider are the principles of pharmacogenomics, a broad-based term that encompasses all genes in the genome that may determine drug response, and pharmacogenetics, the study of how genetics can affect drug action. When pharmacology is applied to patients the usual term is 'therapeutics'.

Pharmacokinetics: The effect of the body on the drug

This is how the body acts on the drug. As far as the body system is concerned, medicines are foreign agents and the aim is to destroy and eliminate them. Pharmacokinetics considers the underlying processes of absorption, distribution, metabolism and elimination. These can be affected by the route of administration, the patient's age, health and many other factors. Whether the medicine is taken orally, is injected, is presented as a patch or as a suppository, absorption into the systemic circulation is a very important phase. The different routes will have a different set of characteristics as far as getting the medicine to the right place in the right concentration and to be there for the right amount of time.

Distribution is the next phase in getting the medicine to the right place. If we consider an oral tablet, then it needs to break down in the stomach and be absorbed across the wall of the small intestine, where most drugs are absorbed. It passes to the liver via the hepatic portal vein where the drug can be metabolised wholly or partially. Metabolites and active drugs will pass into the systemic circulation where they are further distributed, usually bound to circulating proteins in the plasma. As any active drug passes through the liver again it is further metabolised and made water-soluble so it can be eliminated in urine. Any drug that was not absorbed initially will be removed in the faeces.

Terminology in pharmacokinetics

Before we look at each of the four phases in turn, we will look at some terminology that you will come across as you read more. The definitions are given more fully with an example in the glossary.

Bioavailability: This is the proportion of any given drug that reaches the systemic circulation.

Half-life: This is the time taken to reduce the plasma concentration to half of its original value. See the glossary for an example.

Therapeutic index: The therapeutic index of a drug is the ratio of the dose that produces toxicity to the dose that produces a clinically desired or effective response. It is the difference between doing nothing and being toxic. See the glossary for more detail.

Different dosage forms

Activity 6.1

Think about your practice and the prescriptions you have written or have seen. Make a list of the different ways medicines can be given to patients.

Response 6.1 below shows different routes of administration.

Response 6.1 Dosage forms and routes of administration

Oral – *capsules, tablets, liquid medicines swallowed. Tablets can be sugar coated, enteric coated, film coated or uncoated. They can also be sustained release naturally or manufactured that way. Enteric coatings protect the tablet from being destroyed by the acid in the stomach, the coating being removed in the alkaline medium of the small intestine prior to absorption.*

Sublingual – under the tongue

Buccal – kept in the mouth between the lip and the gum

Skin – topical agents such as creams and ointments or via Patches

Rectal – suppositories or creams and ointments

Vaginal – pessaries or simple applications to the surface

Eye drops

Nasal drops and sprays

Inhalation

Injections
- Intravenous
- Intramuscular
- Subcutaneous
- Intrathecal
- Intravitreal: injected into the back of the eye, which is the vitreous cavity.

The four phases of pharmacokinetics

Absorption

In order for any medicine to have a systemic effect it needs to be absorbed and be able to reach the site of action such as receptors inside cells or on cell surfaces. The drug must pass into the circulation to be further distributed. Absorption can be supported by changing the dosage form or by altering the physicochemical properties of the medicine. Medicines need to be fat-soluble to pass across the intestine wall and into the hepatic portal vein. Some chemicals such as vitamin B12 require a carrier to get them across the intestine wall; this is usually called an intrinsic factor. If a patient does not have an intrinsic factor, they cannot absorb vitamin B12 which has a serious effect on red blood cells. Vitamin B12 deficiency is also called cobalamin deficiency. These patients receive regular cobalamin in injection form, removing the need for absorption across the intestine.

Question 6.1

There are occasions when you do not want the drug to be absorbed. When might this be?

Answer 6.1

In patients with C Difficile the problem is in the gut and so you want a potent local-acting drug. The first line drug of choice is the water-soluble antimicrobial vancomycin. The oral formulation is minimally absorbed into the systemic circulation. However, potentially toxic concentrations of vancomycin have been noted in patients with impaired renal function. Systemically, vancomycin is used to treat serious infections such as peritonitis or severe diabetic foot infection.

Some patient characteristics may affect absorption such as gastric emptying or excessive acid production. Similarly, disorders of the GI tract may prevent absorption. If the speed of gastric emptying is increased drugs will enter the small intestine, where most drugs are absorbed more rapidly. If it is delayed, the acid in the stomach can have the effect of destroying some drugs. In patients with, for example, diarrhoea, gut motility is increased and drugs have less time in the small intestine to be absorbed. Other drugs and food can also affect absorption. Antacids which contain heavy metals such as aluminium or magnesium, or milk, which contains calcium, can form insoluble chelates with some medicines such as tetracyclines and prevent their absorption.

Activity 6.2

Look at the BNF section 'Cautionary and advisory labels', which you'll find at the back of the formulary if you are using the hard copy or under the title online. The relevant label numbers are 5, 6, 7, or 23. Now look up ampicillin in the BNF monographs. Under the dosage form oral suspension and capsules you will see that the cautionary labels are numbers 5 and 23. Check what these are by referring to the table in the BNF. Both advise they should be taken on an empty stomach (an hour before or two hours after food) and care is needed if giving antacids.

Distribution

Once in the small intestine, where most drugs are absorbed, the drug passes to the liver via the hepatic portal vein where it is partly metabolised and after metabolism is distributed around the body, usually attached to proteins, frequently albumin. It is important to note that only free drug in the plasma can have a biological effect. Drugs attached to proteins cannot act. However, as the free drug is metabolised in the plasma or attaches to receptors more drug is released from the proteins and becomes active so an equilibrium is maintained until all the active drug is used up. Many drugs are highly protein-bound; if there is any change in the level of protein or competition for protein-binding sites more active drug could be available. If the drug is over 90 per cent protein-bound, small changes or competitive action could have an important effect. For example, warfarin is highly protein-bound (more than 95 per cent) so changes in the amount of protein, for example, in malnutrition or chronic liver disease could have serious consequences as more of the free warfarin would be available.

Metabolism

At first pass, where the absorbed drug molecules have passed across the intestinal wall and have reached the liver via the hepatic portal vein, the main part of metabolism begins to take place. There are two main phases where the body attempts to make the molecules inactive. Both phases decrease the lipophilicity (fat solubility needed to pass across cell walls) of the drug making it more hydrophilic (water-soluble) and thus easier for elimination in the urine.

Phase I reactions are where atoms or molecules are added to the drug molecules. The reactions are oxidation, reduction and hydrolysis by addition of oxygen or removal of hydrogen. The oxidative reactions typically involve a cytochrome P450 monooxygenase which we will discuss later. Although the aim of this is to make the chemical inactive, it generally has the opposite effect, making the 'metabolite' more reactive. Many drugs we have now would be called 'prodrugs' in that they are made into active substances by this process of metabolism.

Phase II reactions are usually known as conjugation reactions – for example, with glucuronic acid, sulfonates (commonly known as sulfation), glutathione or amino acids. They are usually detoxicating in nature. Adding an acetyl group, for example, makes the drug molecules inactive. Some of your patients will be fast or slow acetylators which means they deactivate the molecules of drug slower or faster than normal. This can have a major effect on the activity of the drug given. Some of the inactivated metabolites from the liver may be stored initially in the gall bladder and released back into the gut with bile where they can be reactivated by bacteria in the gut; this is called enterohepatic circulation. The oral contraceptive is an example of this.

The most important enzyme in metabolism in the liver is cytochrome P450. Interactions can occur if any of the isomers of this enzyme are enhanced or inhibited.

Enzyme-inducing drugs

One of your patients is currently taking an effective medicine but you need to give a second drug for a different condition or to enhance the first. If the second drug is an enzyme-inducing drug it will enhance the production of liver enzymes which break down drugs so there is a faster rate of drug breakdown and the first drug will not be as effective as it had been. A larger dose of the affected drug will need to be given to get the same clinical effect.

Examples of enzyme-inducing drugs are shown in **Box 6.1**.

Box 6.1 Enzyme-inducing drugs

- Phenytoin
- Phenobarbitone
- Carbamazepine
- Rifampicin
- Griseofulvin
- Chronic alcohol intake
- Smoking

Enzyme-inhibiting drugs

These inhibit the enzymes which break down drugs in the liver which leads to a decreased rate of drug breakdown and therefore a smaller dose of affected drug is needed to produce the same clinical effect. Examples of these are shown in **Box 6.2**.

Box 6.2   Enzyme inhibitors

Erythromycin	Oral contraceptives
Ciprofloxacin	Sodium valproate
Metronidazole	Cimetidine
Chloramphenicol	Omeprazole

Sulphonamides	Calcium channel blockers
Acute alcohol	Amiodarone
Allopurinol	Dextropropoxyphene
Phenylbutazone	Fluconazole
Isoniazid	

A detailed significance of both of these phenomena is beyond the scope of this short book but any of the textbooks of pharmacology mentioned at the end of this section will give you further details.

Elimination

Metabolites are eventually eliminated via the kidney as they become more water-soluble.

Reading Chapter 8 about different groups of patients and how they may deal with drugs differently is important. You know that as people age their kidney mass and fat levels will alter in many cases but not all. As a rule of thumb after the age of 30 years, creatinine clearance reduces by 8mL/min with every decade, in two-thirds of the population. We measure creatinine clearance as a proxy to kidney function. Creatinine is a waste product that comes from the normal wear and tear on muscles of the body. Everyone has creatinine in their bloodstream. The relatively constant rate of production of creatinine in individual patients together with almost exclusive glomerular filtration means that creatinine clearance (CrCl) should reflect glomerular filtration rate (GFR) and therefore kidney function (see also Chapter 8). Older people, neonates and patients with acute or chronic renal impairment are all likely to have altered renal function.

You need to be particularly careful when prescribing drugs which are renally eliminated. Such drugs include antibiotics, beta blockers and diuretics. Also, caution is needed with drugs that have a narrow therapeutic index such as lithium and, in particular, with drugs that may further reduce renal function, such as NSAIDs.

Pharmacodynamics: The effect of the drug on the body

Drugs work in a number of ways including acting on specific proteins on cell membranes called receptors, blocking the action of specific enzymes, inhibiting cell transport mechanisms and acting directly on invading organisms.

Receptors

As an example, we will consider histamine receptors. Histamine has two main receptors that can be blocked independently or non-specifically. Histamine is a naturally occurring chemical in the body which is released when, for example, pollen is released from grasses and trees and is inhaled. It binds to a histamine receptor, and you get the characteristic runny nose and itchy eyes we call hayfever. Incidentally, by acting on both histamine receptors, the stomach also produces more acid though it will be the other consequences that you are more likely to notice.

An understanding of the different histamine receptors and the development of specific histamine 1 and 2 receptor 'blockers' (known as antagonists) was a relatively recent development, but they have become one of the mainstays of our prescribing. Think about those with severe indigestion or hiatus hernia where they have pain from stomach acid in the stomach or after it has moved into the lower part of the oesophagus. You could recommend an antacid but histamine H_2 receptor blockers are much more efficient and the effect lasts much longer. Another time when you will consider these drugs is when the patient is taking something that may cause irritation of the stomach lining and potentially lead to ulceration. You need something to slow down or stop the acid production in the stomach. Again, specific H_2 receptor antagonists will do this.

Activity 6.3

Find the section in the BNF about H_2 receptor antagonists. See how many there are?

- Cimetidine
- Famotidine
- Nizatidine
- Ranitidine

Notice how all end in 'dine', whereas the brand names are all very different.

Histamine and antihistamine drugs

The older non-specific antihistamines such as diphenhydramine or chlorphenamine can cross the blood–brain barrier so while they are blocking the histamine release as a response to pollen on the nose and eyes they can also block one of the other functions of histamines, which is the role they play in regulating sleep and wakefulness. The older antihistamines cross the blood–brain barrier significantly more than the newer ones. They block the H_1 receptors in the brain. This disruption of the action of histamines in the brain results in drowsiness. This can be a useful action of the antihistamines if you are taking them for sleeplessness due, for example, to itch.

Another important receptor reacts to adrenaline. Adrenaline speeds up the heart and makes it pump harder, it constricts arteries and therefore increases blood pressure. It dilates the bronchioles and opens the airways ready for 'fight or flight'. Drugs that act on the adrenaline receptors and stimulate an action are called adrenergic receptor *agonists*. Salbutamol acts on the beta 2 receptors in the bronchioles causing them to dilate. Older, less specific drugs could dilate the bronchioles but also speed up the heart and increase the blood pressure.

Drugs that function as *antagonists* to adrenaline such as metoprolol and carvedilol block the receptors on the heart and blood vessels which slows the heart and decreases the blood pressure. The older beta blockers such as propranolol also affected the bronchioles, causing them to constrict, and should always be avoided in asthma. Newer more specific beta 1 receptor blockers are reasonably well tolerated in asthma but there are many other antihypertensives that could be considered first.

You will be able to find out much more about receptors and how drugs act as agonists and antagonists in standard pharmacology texts mentioned at the end of this section.

Drugs that inhibit enzymes

In the initial section on pharmacokinetics, we mentioned enzyme inducers and inhibitors in relation to drug metabolism. One enzyme inhibitor we will look at blocks the cyclooxygenase enzymes and is used in musculoskeletal conditions to prevent inflammation and pain.

Inflammation is a bodily action that is important when the body suffers a trauma such as when you bang your thumb with a hammer, or in rheumatoid arthritis, an autoimmune, inflammatory disease. The enzyme which acts to produce the inflammatory reaction and pain is called cyclooxygenase or COX. It is known that there are at least two isomers COX 1 and COX 2, and it has been postulated that there is a COX 3 which is possibly where paracetamol acts.

The non-specific NSAIDs such as ibuprofen, block the production of prostaglandins and therefore inflammation but they act on both COX 1 and COX 2. By this action the pain is addressed as the inflammation can be controlled, but by blocking COX 1 other actions are set in motion such as a reduction in the stomach-protecting mucous which could lead to ulceration of the stomach. Specific COX 2 enzyme blockers have been developed but they have their own side-effects which have limited their use in practice.

There are other enzyme-blocking drugs such as angiotensin-converting enzyme (ACE) inhibitors which can be used to help reduce blood pressure, but this is beyond the scope of this short chapter. Homeostasis is the body's way of maintaining a state of balance among all the body systems; one of these is blood pressure. Angiotensin is a peptide hormone and vasoconstrictor which increases blood pressure. If this becomes out of balance blood pressure will rise. By blocking the conversion of angiotensin 1 to angiotensin 2, blood pressure can be reduced. The action is, as with other systems, not totally specific and the blocking of angiotensin 1 to 2 also has the effect of blocking the breakdown of bradykinin. This can have an effect of making the bronchioles more sensitive and can cause an irritating cough. If this becomes a problem for your patient, potentially leading to non-adherence, you could consider angiotensin II receptor antagonists such as irbesartan which act directly on the angiotensin 2 receptor and do not affect bradykinin.

Drugs that affect cell transport

The example we are using is that of the calcium channel blockers. They are not antagonists as they do not compete for receptor sites; they block the transport of, in this case, calcium ions which prevent the passage of electrical stimuli – in turn, this stops whatever reaction was being undertaken. In a nerve cell this might be to prevent nerve conduction when using local anaesthetics; in the case of calcium channel blockers, they act on the cell membrane of vascular smooth muscle, in other words on blood vessels, preventing contraction and therefore are used to reduce blood pressure.

Pharmacogenomics and personalised medicine

Principles of pharmacogenomics and pharmacogenetics

Pharmacogenetics is the study of how genetics can affect pharmacokinetics and pharmacodynamics and therefore how drugs will have their effect in an individual. More recently, the term 'pharmacogenomics' has been introduced. The word pharmacogenomics links pharmacology to genetics and is the study of how a person's genes can affect their response to drugs. Pharmacogenomics is used to help develop effective medications based on a person's genetic make-up.

While pharmacogenetics is largely used in relation to individual genes, pharmacogenomics is a broader-based term that encompasses all genes in the genome that may determine the patient's response to a drug; both terms are often used interchangeably.

As you will see in Chapter 8, there is a variation in the response to drugs based on a number of factors such as age, gender and race. For example, drug elimination is less efficient in older people where drugs can have prolonged or greater effects. The half-life of benzodiazepines such as diazepam can increase with age and accumulation can occur if doses remain the same. The plasma half-life of benzodiazepines can increase, which is important as there can be an accumulation if the dose is maintained at normal levels (Ritter et al., 2020).

Chapter 8 explores the need to be particularly careful in prescribing for different patient groups such as older people, neonates, children and pregnant women, and describes changes in aspects of pharmacology in different patient groups. Benzodiazepines can produce more confusion but less sedation in older people and this could be misinterpreted as age-related memory impairment rather than to the drug accumulation.

Genetic Variation On Drug Responsiveness

Mutations can be inherited when they affect the sperm or egg. Acquired mutations are not present at birth and are not passed on to offspring.

Some useful further reading

There are many excellent books on pharmacology and therapeutics. Some are said to be geared to nurses, others to pharmacists and others to the general market. As our understanding of the principles of pharmacology develops, it is best you look at various volumes to see which you prefer.

Glossary of terms and examples used in pharmacokinetics

Bioavailability. This is the proportion of any given drug that reaches the systemic circulation. If you give an intravenous injection, 100 per cent will reach the circulation; in contrast, if taken orally or via any other route, some will be destroyed before it reaches the plasma. Bioavailability is usually given as a number from 0–1 where 1 is 100 per cent.

What do you think bioavailability could be affected by? See **Box 6.3**. It is important to note that the effect may be to slow down or speed up the drug reaching the systemic circulation but this may not affect its bioavailability. It is the proportion that reaches the systemic circulation, not how long it takes.

Box 6.3

Dosage form may delay or speed up reaching the systemic circulation as this will affect the absorption.

Dissolution and absorption of the drug. If absorption is affected negatively, then the bioavailability will be lower.

Route of administration. Injections versus oral route will affect the time but not always the proportion reaching the systemic circulation.

Stability of the drug in the GI tract (if oral route). If unstable then the bioavailability of drugs presented by the oral route will be reduced. Changes may be needed either in the route of administration or in the physical form if oral is needed – for example, adding an enteric coating.

Extent of drug metabolism before reaching systemic circulation. If the drug is highly metabolised, less will reach the circulation and the bioavailability will be reduced.

Presence of food/drugs in GI tract. This can affect absorption and, in some cases, prevent it but in others it may enhance absorption.

Question 6.2

Half-life example

Say a patient is taking a drug and has a toxic blood level of 16mg/L and the blood level you want is 2mg/L. You know the drug half-life is eight hours. How long will it take for the blood level to fall back to the level you want?

Answer 6.2

- 16mg to 8mg = 8 hours
- 8mg to 4mg = 8 hours
- 4mg to 2mg = 8 hours
- *Total: 24 hours*

Therapeutic index

The therapeutic index of a drug is the ratio of the dose that produces toxicity to the dose that produces a clinically desired or effective response. It is the difference between doing nothing and being toxic.

You obviously want the dose to be effective but not toxic. Some drugs have a very wide therapeutic index and normal doses are unlikely to cause problems but there are many drugs where the therapeutic index is narrow and dosing must be very carefully controlled. Drugs with a narrow therapeutic index include, for example, digoxin, gentamicin, carbamazepine, phenytoin, lithium and theophylline.

Where the therapeutic index is narrow it is important not to increase a dose without careful monitoring. There are two ways of changing the amount of drug in the circulation. One is to increase the dose and the other is to increase the frequency. If the therapeutic index is narrow it may be better to increase the frequency rather than the dose.

For example, a patient maintained in dihydrocodeine at a dose of 30mg every eight hours has breakthrough pain. Increasing the dose to 60mg every eight hours can lead to toxic levels of dihydrocodeine whereas increasing the frequency to every four hours will manage the pain without leading to toxic levels.

This is a rare example but highlights a potential issue.

Antimicrobials: The 'magic bullets'

In the *Competency Framework for All Prescribers* (RPS, 2021), there are several competencies and support statements that need to be considered when prescribing antimicrobials. There are general statements that are important in all aspects of prescribing, including prescribing antimicrobials. For example, Competency 1, Assess the patient, stresses the need for an appropriate clinical assessment; statements 1.7 and 1.10 request relevant investigations. Competency 2, Identify evidence-based treatment options available for clinical decision-making, has a number of general relevant supporting statements and some specific, such as 2.9: 'Considers the wider perspective including the public health issues related to medicines and their use and promoting health'. This will be discussed when we look at antibiotic resistance. Supporting statement 2.10 specifically mentions this: 'Understands antimicrobial resistance and the roles of infection prevention, control and antimicrobial stewardship measures'. All will be discussed in this chapter.

Introduction and history of antimicrobials

Antimicrobials are life-saving drugs used to treat commonly occurring infections; their contributions to improved health outcomes during the 20th century is significant. There is a long history of the use of antimicrobials in treating infections, with some historians recording their use as far back as Egyptian times. Scientists such as Paul Ehrlich and Alexander Fleming were instrumental in identifying the potential for the use of antibiotics and in 1945 Howard Florey and Ernst Chain were awarded the Nobel Prize in medicines for their contributions to the large-scale production of these treatments (Microbiology Society, 2022).

This drug group is vitally important in modern medicine due to the significant benefits not only to an individual's health outcomes, but also to aspects of public health. This is of significance in recent times when growing concerns about global antimicrobial resistance dominate health discourses.

What is an antibiotic?

The terms 'antimicrobial' and 'antibiotic' are often used interchangeably though what they are describing is slightly different. Antimicrobial is an umbrella term that encompasses chemical substances, of natural or synthetic origin, that suppress the growth of, or destroy, micro-organisms including bacteria, fungi, helminths (worms), protozoa and viruses (Waller and Sampson, 2018). Antibiotics specifically refer to those substances that target bacteria.

Antibiotics utilise a variety of mechanisms to stop growth (bacteriostatic) or destroy bacteria (bactericidal). The mechanism depends on the class of antibiotic with three main targets (BSAC, 2018):

- bacterial cell wall or membrane
- synthesis of nucleic acids DNA and RNA
- protein synthesis.

Antibiotics can target bacterial cells without harming human cells due to the cellular make-up; Paul Ehrlich referred to them as 'magic bullets' (Strebhardt and Ullrich, 2008).

You will have seen these drugs used in various ways. For example, they can be used prophylactically, to prevent infection; empirically, when you suspect infection but have not had this confirmed by microbiology; or definitively, when you know the specific pathogen and you can target the treatment precisely. Antibiotics are commonly prescribed, although in recent years there has been a downward trend in their use (Nuffield Trust, 2021) likely linked to safer prescriber initiatives designed to reduce inappropriate antibiotic usage to prevent antimicrobial resistance (NHS England, 2021).

Antimicrobial resistance

Antimicrobial resistance (AMR) is a significant global threat and a serious public health risk which leaves populations vulnerable as antimicrobials used to treat common infections run the risk of becoming ineffective (WHO, 2021a). AMR is predicted to lead to 10 million deaths by 2050; this is exacerbated by a lack of new antimicrobials in the pipeline (DHSC, 2019).

The advent of AMR was known from the very beginning: 'The thoughtless person playing with penicillin treatment is morally responsible for the death of the man who succumbs to infection with the penicillin-resistant organism' (Sir Alexander Fleming, 1945, quoted in Nogrady, 2016). AMR occurs when bacteria, viruses, fungi and parasites change over time and no longer respond to medicines, making infections harder to treat and increasing the risk of disease spread, severe illness and death (WHO, 2021a).

Some AMR is naturally occurring (intrinsic) resistance, meaning the antibiotic was never sensitive to begin with. However, 'man-made' drivers such as overuse and misuse of antimicrobials, coupled with poor sanitation and hygiene, as well as limited access in some countries to vaccinations and appropriate treatment has resulted in growth of acquired resistance (BSAC, 2018). This is where the original species was sensitive and the organism has developed resistance to the antibiotic.

Some mechanisms by which organisms have rendered antimicrobials inactive include:

a. inactivation of the antibiotic;

b. active efflux (the process whereby, molecules including antimicrobials are transported outside the cell and away from the site of action);

c. changing the target;

d. limiting uptake.

(Reygaert, 2018)

These mechanisms can be passed from bacteria to bacteria by a process called conjugation, where the genetic material responsible for the resistant mechanism is transferred. When antibiotics are prescribed these 'mutant' bacteria survive and can result in treatment failure. Inactivation of the antibiotics by producing enzymes which break down antibiotics is commonly seen with beta-lactams, a wide group that includes penicillins and cephalosporins, where the enzyme beta-lactamase breaks down beta-lactam antibiotics.

AMR has been around forever so why bother now?

As a prescriber, you need to be aware that rates of AMR are increasing globally and are linked to antimicrobial consumption (DHSC, 2019). There is also a known economic cost; patients with resistant infections often need treatment for longer and with more expensive antibiotics, with an estimated cumulative cost of AMR thought to be US $100 trillion by 2050 (DHSC, 2019) The need for you, as a nurse prescriber, to develop safer prescribing practices is imperative.

You are probably thinking, how am I going to stop this? Thankfully, as a nurse prescriber you are in the perfect position to play a role by using antimicrobials only when appropriate, in accordance with guidelines and with up-to-date patient information such as allergies, cultures and sensitivities. Following infection prevention and control measures (see later) and educating both yourself and patients on conditions that do not require antibiotics or are self-limiting are also important.

Antimicrobial stewardship

You will have heard of antimicrobial stewardship but what exactly is it? There are various definitions including 'an organisational or healthcare-system-wide approach to promoting and monitoring judicious use of antimicrobials to preserve their future effectiveness' (NICE, 2015a).

But what does stewardship mean in practice?

Key point

If an antibiotic is necessary, antimicrobial stewardship means using the optimum dose, duration and selection of antibiotics, to treat or prevent infection, while ensuring minimal toxicity and impact on resistance. In even more simplified terms, it is the right antibiotic, at the right dose, for the right duration, for that patient for that specific infection. Following this stewardship mantra should help protect antimicrobials and prevent AMR.

Diagnosis

As prescribers your first task is to agree a diagnosis and if an antimicrobial would be appropriate using an appropriate clinical assessment (Competency 1, Assess the patient, RPS, 2021), including history taking, physical examination and imaging, such as X-rays, MRIs, alongside the use of diagnostic tests – for example, sputum, urine, or blood cultures – to help support the decision-making process and confirm the diagnosis. Point of care (POC) testing is a prime example where having the right diagnostic tests and results rapidly can help to reduce prescribing of antibiotics (Cooke, 2015; Mantzourani et al., 2022); with care closer to home identified in the *NHS Long Term Plan*, use of POC testing in places such as community pharmacies and GP practices is important to achieve this (NHS England, 2019). Examples include urine dipsticks, which, although best avoided in those over 65 due to asymptomatic bacteriuria being more common, can be useful in most age groups. Others such as influenza and COVID POC tests can help to cohort and isolate patients to aid with infection prevention and control.

Some infections can be self-limiting in nature, whereby they resolve of their own accord over time and simple supportive measures such as hydration and pain relief can be applied. This often occurs in immunocompetent patients, where the body's natural immune defence can cope. Sore throats are often self-limiting, with the majority caused by respiratory viruses (NICE, 2018b). A recent meta-analysis found that 82 per cent of participants who took placebo, or received no treatment were symptom-free at one week, with antibiotics providing no or very modest benefit (Spinks et al., 2021). While a small reduction in symptoms can be seen, this must be weighed against the potential adverse effects of antibiotics as well as the impact on resistance.

It is also important to consider differential diagnosis, severe infections or when the patient is deteriorating. For example, sore throat is a symptom of scarlet fever, a streptococcal infection where a typical scarlatina-type rash develops due to presence of the bacterial toxin. It is more common in children; a useful traffic light system has been produced to help identify those at risk (NICE, 2015b) which leads us nicely on to …

The right patient

Patient-specific factors that need to be taken into consideration include, allergies, age, severity of symptoms, comorbidities, immunosuppression and previous antibiotic use. A child with a sore throat and fever is likely to require antibiotics, and further assessment (NICE, 2015b) compared to an afebrile adult with mild symptoms, who may manage with supportive measures.

Establishing information about the patient's allergy history is vital. Patients with penicillin allergies receive less effective and more costly antibiotics, are associated with longer stays in hospital and therefore increased risk of infections with methicillin-resistant Staphylococcus aureus (MRSA) and Clostridioides difficile (Wanat et al., 2021). Around 10 per cent of the population has an allergy to penicillin listed on their GP records, but only 5 per cent of these have a true penicillin allergy (NICE, 2018a). There is also a 10 per cent risk of reaction to other penicillin-like antibiotics such as cephalosporins and carbapenems.

Allergies fall into two categories: immediate onset, where urticaria, anaphylaxis, bronchospasm and angioedema are present – these are Immunoglobulin E (IgE)-mediated and tend to occur within an hour; and delayed or Immunoglobulin G (IgG) reactions, which can cause maculopapular or morbilliform rashes, with Steven Johnson syndrome, a serious example of which can occur with co-trimoxazole (Blumenthal et al., 2019). Over time IgE reactions can wane resulting in no reaction when re-challenged. Around 10 per cent of the UK population has a reported penicillin allergy, but only around 20 per cent of these will be truly allergic (BMJ, 2017). Given the burden of AMR, work is ongoing to develop pathways and tools to help review these patients and aid the removal of spurious allergies labels.

The right antibiotic

Choosing an antibiotic should not be a lucky dip. Different antibiotics cover different bacteria, primarily due to the differences in the cell structure between the two main bacterial groups: gram-positive, such as Staphylococcus aureus, and gram-negative, Escherichia coli bacteria. This difference means some antibiotics which target the cell wall – for example, glycopeptides, are not effective against any gram-negative bacteria.

You might say: 'But I can't know every bacterium each antibiotic covers.' You are right! That is where guidelines help. NICE produce guidelines for common infections (NICE, 2022b) as part of the UK strategy on AMR, along with other initiatives such as the TARGET toolkits for primary care (RCGP, 2019). Guidelines ensure that the most common bacteria are covered – for example, skin and soft tissue infections such as cellulitis are predominantly caused by staphylococcus and streptococcus species (Fulton et al., 2005). Conversely urine infections are associated with gram-negative organisms, mainly E. coli. However, it is also important to refer to local guidelines where available; this is due to local resistance patterns. For example, the rate of E. coli which is resistant to ciprofloxacin in one trust is 12.0 per cent, while a neighbouring trust reported a 24.0 per cent resistance (UKHSA, 2023).

Initial treatment will be empiric – that is, based on your experience, knowledge and the patient's description. This *Start Smart: Then Focus* model is another toolkit to help tackle AMR primarily used for secondary care (PHE, 2015), but applicable across any healthcare domain. As the causative bacteria may not be known, a broad-spectrum antibiotic is likely to be chosen which will cover most common bacteria, 'starting smart'. This can then be rationalised once and, if microbiological diagnosis is available, a more 'focused' approach with narrow-spectrum antibiotics can be used. However, sometimes consultation with microbiology specialists, such as antimicrobial pharmacists, is required in cases of resistance.

The choice of antibiotic then must be linked back to the patient, considering other medications and comorbidities, as well as ability to take oral antibiotics. First, drug-drug interactions are important. The penicillins interact with very few medications, but macrolides (clarithromycin, erythromycin) and quinolones (ciprofloxacin, levofloxacin) are known inhibitors of Cytochrome P450 enzymes. Therefore, existing medication that the patient takes that may be metabolised via these enzymes can accumulate within the body, potentially causing increased adverse effects or toxicity.

Absorption of many antibiotics can be affected by food – for example, flucloxacillin should be taken on an empty stomach, either before food or two hours after (BNF, 2023). This can be difficult for some patients, especially as the dosing is every six hours. Tetracyclines (doxycycline, oxytetracycline) can chelate (bind to) ion salts, such as calcium, iron, magnesium and zinc, so foods or medication including these should be two hours before or after taking a tetracycline (BNF, 2023). Linezolid, which is a MOA-inhibitor used to treat skin and soft skin infections, can cause a hypertensive crisis when tyramine-rich foods are consumed alongside it; examples include mature cheese, soya sauce, yeast extracts and undistilled alcoholic beverages (Pfizer, 2018).

While having an alcoholic drink while feeling unwell might not be the priority, a few may have been in the situation: a best friend's wedding, birthday parties etc. It is unlikely that drinking in moderation will have a detrimental effect when taking antibiotics. However, side-effects such as dizziness and nausea may be made worse (NHS, 2022a). Metronidazole is one antibiotic where consuming alcohol should be avoided. This is due to a Disulfiram-type reaction. Disulfiram is a medication to help keep people abstinent; it works by inhibiting the breakdown of alcohol, leading to accumulation resulting in diaphoresis, palpitations, facial flushing, nausea, vertigo, hypotension and tachycardia (Stokes and Abdijadid, 2022).

Thinking about the patient's other characteristics is important; a frail elderly patient with chronic kidney disease may require different antibiotics due to their renal function, while some antibiotics, such as ertapenem and ciprofloxacin, can lower seizure threshold and therefore should be avoided in those patients with conditions that may predispose them to seizures.

Activity 6.4

Interactions: Clarithromycin inhibits the metabolism of statins, resulting in increased concentrations of the statin in the body. This increases the risk of rhabdomyolysis. How would you negate this?

Response 6.4

When using a short course of clarithromycin, omitting the statin for the duration of the antibiotic would negate this reaction. If the duration is more long term, such as prophylaxis of cellulitis, consideration as to the choice of antibiotic would be required. The other option here would be to consider changing the anti-lipid therapy if a change in antibiotic was not appropriate.

The right dose and duration

The minimum inhibitory concentration (MIC) is the lowest concentration required to prevent growth of a bacteria in vitro. These readings are compared with clinical breakpoints, which are the minimum concentration at which the organism's growth is *unlikely* to be inhibited by a specific antibiotic at a set dose (Hand and Joseph, 2021). If the MIC is below this breakpoint, it is considered sensitive; if close to the breakpoint, intermediate; and if above it is considered resistant. The breakpoints are set by the European Committee on Antimicrobial Susceptibility Testing (EUCAST), which tests thousands of 'drug-bug' combinations (Hand and Joseph, 2021), helps local, national and international review and sets dosing.

The doses of antimicrobials recommended in the BNF should ensure that these are met for most bacteria; however, patient factors such as severity of infection, weight, comorbidities and resistance may require dose changes. For example, UK Clinical Pharmacy Association (UKCPA, 2013) provides useful information on dosing in obese adults who are critically ill and the Specialist Pharmacy Service (SPS) provides information on dosing in obese children (Burgess, 2021).

Guidelines provide recommended doses and course length, with this being the shortest effective course. A cross-sectional study found that 1.3 million days of treatment were given beyond the recommended duration (Pouwels et al., 2019); clearly this will add further fuel to the AMR fire and the implications that come with this, including an estimated cost of US $4.6 million in 2017 in the United States alone (Nelson et al., 2021). Therefore, being familiar with recommended durations and changes to guidance is important. A recent article suggests a move away from 'complete the course' to 'take exactly as prescribed'. We discussed target selection above, but the main reasoning behind this suggestion is collateral selection. This occurs when other bacteria that may be living harmlessly in our gut or on our skin and which are not the cause of the infection develop resistance to the antibiotic; key examples include MRSA and extended spectrum β-lactamase producing Enterobacteriaceae (ESBLs) (Llewelyn et al., 2017).

Activity 6.5

Look at the TARGET toolkit for primary care for UTI (RCGP, 2019). Use this to reflect on a case you may have been involved in. Would you do anything differently this time round?

Factors affecting choices of treatments

Case Study 6.1

Mrs Grant is a 70-year-old female who presents to clinic complaining of pain on urination with an increased frequency, including during the night.

Allergies: none

She takes the following:

Aspirin 75mg daily

Atorvastatin 20mg daily

Ramipril 2.5mg daily
- What is the likely diagnosis and potential differential diagnosis?
- What tests/investigations would you order?
- What course of action would you suggest? If you suggest an antibiotic, provide a dose and duration using the BNF and appropriate guidelines.

Case Study 6.1 Responses (NICE, 2022c)

What is the likely diagnosis and differential diagnosis?

Likely lower UTI – two or more symptoms consistent with UTI, dysuria, nocturia and pain on urination.

Differential diagnosis

Red Flags – such as haematuria, loin pain, rigors, nausea, vomiting and altered mental state which could indicate sepsis or upper UTI.

Upper UTI – given pain, would need further questioning around this.

Depending on results of investigations other diagnosis could be sexually transmitted infections – chlamydia, contact dermatitis, malignancies.

What tests/investigations would you order?

Assessment of the patient including vital signs, temperature, blood pressure, heart and respiratory rate to help identify systemic illness.

A urine culture should always be sent in cases who are over 65 with a suspected UTI.

Urine dipstick should be avoided in this age group as often they have asymptomatic bacteriuria, and a dipstick is therefore unreliable. Urine dipsticks can still be useful in other patient groups.

Other tests would include:
- white cell count, C-reactive protein (CRP). Procalcitonin (PCT) is a relatively new marker of infection, which is more specific for bacterial infection than CRP. It is useful for identifying systemic infection, but also to rule out bacterial causes due to the high negative predictive value of PCT (Levine et al., 2018);
- urea and electrolytes are helpful to determine the impact on the kidneys and potential severity of the infection. An AKI may suggest more systemic infection and sepsis (UK Sepsis Trust, 2022). It is also useful for dosing of antibiotics.

You may consider requesting an ultrasound of the kidneys, particularly if symptoms of loin pain, suggesting an upper UTI or pyelonephritis.

If a male patient has recurrent UTIs he should be investigated for urological abnormalities – for example, by undertaking an ultrasound of the urinary tract.

What course of action would you suggest? If you suggest an antibiotic, provide a dose and duration using the BNF and appropriate guidelines.

Given Mrs Grant's age she is at increased risk of infection.

Given the current lack of results you would need to revisit previous urine cultures (of which there are none).

Given no previous urine results, antibiotic therapy would need to be empiric.

We need to know what her allergy status is before prescribing: Mrs Grant has no known allergies.

Based on (NICE, 2022a):
- 1st line – Nitrofurantoin 100mg MR BD or 50mg QDS for three days
- 2nd line – Trimethoprim 200mg BD for three days
- 3rd line – Pivmecillinam 400mg Stat then 200mg TDS for three days.

Be aware of local resistance patterns and check local guidelines as the options may differ.

Things to consider in this case:
- if eGFR < 45mL/minute then nitrofurantoin will not be effective;
- potential increased risk of hyperkalaemia with trimethoprim and ramipril at the same time.

Severity of infection

This can often be determined when you carry out the clinical assessment at the consultation, as well as by microbiology results; however, positive microbiology may not be obtained in all cases. A recent study found that five bacteria, Staphylococcus aureus, Escherichia coli, Streptococcus pneumoniae, Klebsiella pneumoniae and Pseudomonas aeruginosa, were responsible for 54·9 per cent of deaths in 2019, with lower respiratory, bloodstream infections and intra-abdominal infections the three main conditions caused by these bacteria (Ikuta et al., 2029).

Clinical assessment, patient history (including procedures, travel and other past medical history) and imaging such as X-rays and MRIs are vital pieces in the infection jigsaw. Tools such as National Early Warning Score (NEWS) (RCP, 2017) are helpful to assess severity of illness, using six commonly measured parameters (see **Box 6.4**).

Box 6.4

In NEWS2, the latest version of National Early Warning Score, the six parameters are:

- respiratory rate
- oxygen saturation
- systolic blood pressure
- pulse rate
- level of consciousness or new confusion
- temperature.

Although not specifically related to infection, NEWS2 is a standardised assessment of severity of illness, identifying serious illness or deterioration to trigger the appropriate clinical response. Sepsis should be considered in any patient with a NEWS2 score of 5. Sepsis is the body's overreaction to infection or injury. This overreaction can lead to organ failure and even death (UK Sepsis Trust, 2022). Those who present with any one of the red flags should be started immediately on the sepsis 6 pathway. Sepsis Red Flags (UK Sepsis Trust, 2022)

- Acute confusional state
- Systolic B.P ≤ 90 mmHg (or drop >40 from normal)
- Heart rate > 130 per minute
- Respiratory rate ≥ 25 per minute
- Needs oxygen to keep SpO2 ≥92%
- Non-blanching rash, mottled/ashen/cyanotic

- Not passed urine in last 18 h/Urine Output <0.5mL/kg/hr L
- Lactate ≥2 mmol/l
- Recent chemotherapy

Applying the Sepsis 6 bundle within the first hour following recognition of sepsis has been shown to greatly increase a patient's chances of survival. Part of this bundle includes fluids, oxygen (if required), but also administration of intravenous antibiotics. However, blood cultures should ideally be taken prior to antibiotic treatment starting, to increase the chances of a positive result.

When infection is suspected, markers such as white cell count (WCC) and C-reactive protein (CRP) will be requested along with relevant microbiological samples such as sputum, blood and urine cultures and wound swabs. Procalcitonin (PCT) has become another useful inflammatory marker. As a precursor of the hormone calcitonin produced by thyroid and lungs, under normal metabolic conditions PCT is undetectable in blood. However, in response to pro-inflammatory causes, mainly, but not limited to bacterial infection, PCT is produced by numerous other cells. This results in increased levels of PCT, especially in severe sepsis and systemic infection. The value of PCT is seen the most when de-escalating and ceasing antimicrobials, where viral or non-infective causes may be present such as flu or exacerbations of asthma. As with any other biomarker, interpretation must be made with reference to the patient.

Other non-specific infection-related blood tests such as creatinine, urea, lactate and liver function can all help to understand how well the body is functioning in response to the infection. In sepsis these tests are vital to identify any organ dysfunction. Lactate is particularly important in sepsis, as this predicts outcome, with a high lactate resulting in a greater likelihood of critical care admission; the reasoning for this is outside the scope of this chapter.

Infection-specific tools are also used when assessing severity of infection. CURB-65 (Lim et al., 2003), for community-acquired pneumonia, calculates the mortality risk of a patient and therefore the severity of infection. This determines the choice of treatment including oral or intravenous antibiotics. The Duke criteria (from Duke University Medical Center), which is used in conjunction with clinical assessment, helps determine the likelihood of endocarditis as a diagnosis (Li et al., 2000).

Case study 6.2

Four days later Mrs Grant presents to A&E with loin tenderness, dysuria, shivers, shakes, sweats, malaise and vomiting.

- On admission
- Heart rate 120 beats per minute
- Respiratory rate 20 breaths per minute
- Blood pressure 110/70 mmHg
- Temperature 39.1 °C
- Height 1.6m
- She is started on intravenous gentamicin
- Calculate NEWS2 score
- What is the likely diagnosis?
- (Reference ranges from – LTHT, 2023)

Initial bloods
White cell count 17×10^9 /L ($4 - 11 \times 10^9$ /L)
Creatine 170 μmol /L ($49 - 90$ μmol /L)

CRP 100mg/L (< 10mg/L)
Weight 65Kg

Case study 6.2 Responses

NEWS2 score of 5

- 1 for blood pressure
- 2 for temperature
- 2 for heart rate

Diagnosis – Sepsis – likely sepsis of urinary origin.

Sepsis should be considered here as per the NEWS2 score.

Given the patient's previous treatment for a lower UTI, and symptoms of loin tenderness/ dysuria it is most likely to be of urinary cause. Could also be abdominal in origin.

Route

The severity and site of infection will determine the route by which the antibiotic is given. In sepsis the bacterial load is likely to be high and absorption can be affected so intravenous antibiotics are the most reliable. Penetration and the deep-seated nature of some bone or central nervous system infections will often necessitate initial intravenous treatment.

Intravenous antibiotics should be reviewed within 48 hours, and a decision made to see if switch to an oral form is appropriate. The United Kingdom Health Security Agency (UKHSA) has recently published an IV to oral decision aid, which has been developed by gaining a UK-wide consensus (UKHSA, 2022). This national tool is a key aid when reviewing patients on intravenous antibiotics. The tool can be accessed from: www.gov.uk/government/ publications/antimicrobial-intravenous-to-oral-switch-criteria-for-early-switch

If you are the nurse prescriber initiating the IV antibiotic treatment, the review and consideration of oral treatments is a key part of your stewardship role. Although intravenous antibiotics are often thought to be superior as they are 100 per cent bioavailable, some oral antibiotics also achieve this such as linezolid, levofloxacin, ciprofloxacin and clindamycin. Oral antibiotics have been shown to be as effective as intravenous in various infections including bone and joint (Li et al., 2019) and endocarditis (Iversen et al., 2018). Intravenous antibiotics also require intravenous access, which can put the patient at risk of healthcare-acquired infection and phlebitis.

Another good reason to consider the oral route is the impact of intravenous administration on the environment. Compared to oral, intravenous administration has far more impact, with oral administration accounting for 1/45th of the emissions of intravenous paracetamol. Switching a third of these to oral would save around 5 tonnes of carbon dioxide per year, from primary production and waste disposal (Myo et al., 2021). This is around the same with intravenous antibiotics compared with their oral equivalents.

Case study 6.3

Mrs Grant was started on IV gentamicin; a day later her routine blood results came back.

She has grown E. coli in her blood culture sensitive to nitrofurantoin, pivmecillinam, ciprofloxacin and gentamicin.

- On admission
- WCC 17 × 10^9 /L
- CRP 150mg/L
- Creatinine 150 µmol /L

Current bloods
WCC 15 × 10^9 /L (4 – 11 × 10^9 /L)
CRP 100mg/L (< 10mg/L)
Creatinine 240 µmol /L (49 – 90 µmol /L)

Gentamicin level: 3mg/L (pre-dose level) (< 2mg/l).

You are asked when the next dose of gentamicin is due and whether you should give it.

Suggest a regimen for Mrs Grant's antibiotics, including antibiotic, dose and duration.

Case study 6.3 Responses

Various gentamicin regimens are used across the country, with the majority using either 5mg/kg dosing or 7mg/kg (Hartford) dosing.

Before looking at the level itself, check that it has been taken at the correct time:
- 5mg/kg dosing – pre-dose (around four hours before next dose). The level must be below 1mg/L before the next dose can be given.
- 7mg/kg dosing – level is taken six to 14 hours post dose. If this window is missed a random level may be taken. If the level is less than 2mg/l a second dose can be given.

(Garraghan and Fallon, 2015)

As this is a pre-dose level it would be not safe to give due to the risk of toxicity. It is also important to take into consideration renal function.

Renal function

CrCl initially is 28mL/min (25mL/min based on adjusted body weight) and deteriorates to 20mL/min (17mL/min based on adjusted body weight).

There has been a clear jump in creatinine, corresponding to an AKI 1. Given gentamicin is nephrotoxic, this is likely to be as a result of treatment, therefore it would be advisable to cease the gentamicin altogether and consider another agent.

Other options

Nitrofurantoin – requires adequate renal function as antibacterial effect requires renal secretion of drug into urinary tract, therefore should be avoided if eGFR <45 (BNF, 2023).
It should also be avoided in upper UTI/urosepsis due to lack of adequate drugs levels in renal tissue (NICE, 2018c).

Pivmecillinam – no issues with renal function but does not achieve adequate levels in renal tissue therefore should be avoided in upper UTI/urosepsis (NICE, 2018c).

Both these options may have also already been used first line.

Ciprofloxacin – has good oral bioavailability, so oral is as a good as intravenous, if there are no absorption issues. There are, however, several safety issues to be aware of including tendonitis, especially in the older population (BNF, 2023; NICE, 2018c). It would be a risk–benefit and, given we have no further sensitivities, the most suitable option.

Dose: 250–500mg 12 hourly daily for seven days.

Ciprofloxacin also has the added benefit that a duration of seven days treatment is sufficient, when compared to some other options. Courses of other antibiotics range from ten to 14 days (NICE, 2018c).

Adverse effects

Unfortunately, these 'magic bullets' – like all medicines – have side-effects. I am sure you are well versed in the common (1 in 100 to 1 in 10) side-effects of antibiotics, namely nausea, vomiting and diarrhoea (BNF, 2023). We have also touched on allergy and allergic reactions above, with patients commonly labelled penicillin allergic when the majority aren't truly allergic.

Other adverse effects can be related to the narrow therapeutic index of certain antibiotics – for example, nephrotoxicity with glycopeptides – while aminoglycosides can also result in ototoxicity, which is irreversible (Garraghan and Fallon, 2015). In secondary care these two drugs require therapeutic drug monitoring to ensure we reach effective levels to kill the bacteria but also to monitor and prevent toxic levels within the blood.

Some specific side-effects to be aware of (BNF, 2023):

Quinolones: Tendonitis, aortic aneurysm, heart valve regurgitation, QT prolongation, reduce seizure threshold

Clindamycin: Can cause severe diarrhoea – colitis

Linezolid: Blood dyscrasias, requires weekly full blood monitoring for each week of treatment

Penicillin (particularly flucloxacillin, co-amoxiclav and piperacillin/ tazobactam): Liver test derangement. False-positive urinary glucose (if testing for reducing substances)

Prescribing and infection prevention and control

You will have already embedded infection prevention strategies into your everyday practise in order to reduce the risks healthcare-acquired infection transmission. Evidence-based principles of infection prevention and control should also be applied to your prescribing encounters and decisions in order to protect patients (WHO, 2021b). Principles of infection prevention should be applied when undertaking prescribing consultations and assessing patients. You will also need to consider infection prevention when making judgements about suitable treatments in order to minimise the impact of harm associated with AMR and 'superbugs'.

Infections caused by 'superbugs' have a significant impact on patient morbidity and mortality; they are associated with significant financial costs to the NHS. They pose a significant global threat to health and mitigation is essential to maintain the integrity of current evidence-based treatment pathways. For more information about superbugs, please see Appendix 2.

Summary

As you have seen, pharmacokinetics is the way the body acts on medicines and pharmacodynamics which is how the medicine acts on the body to have its effect. Two newer areas are considered which are pharmacogenomics and pharmacogenetics.

Infection control, including interventions such as screening, reporting and infection prevention and control strategies, is important. Antimicrobials are life-saving drugs used to treat commonly occurring infections and their contributions to improved health outcomes during the 20th century is significant. However, antimicrobial resistance (AMR) is a significant global threat and a serious public health risk which leaves populations vulnerable as antimicrobials used to treat common infections run the risk of becoming ineffective.

A key learning point is that of antimicrobial stewardship which means that if an antibiotic is necessary, the optimum dose, duration and selection of antibiotic is used to treat or prevent infection, while ensuring minimal toxicity and impact on resistance.

Further reading

Downie, G., Mackenzie, J., Williams, A. and Milne, C. 2007. *Pharmacology and Medicines Management for Nurses*. 4th ed. Edinburgh: Churchill Livingstone.

Golan, D.E. 2016. *Principles of Pharmacology: The Pathophysiologic Basis of Drug Therapy*. Baltimore, MD: Lippincott Williams and Wilkins.

Neal, M.J. 2020. *Medical Pharmacology at a Glance*. 9th ed. Chichester: Wiley-Blackwell.

Ritter, J.A.M., Flower, R., Henderson, G., Loke, Y.K., MacEwan, D.J. and Rang, H.P. 2020. *Rang and Dale's Pharmacology*. 9th ed. Edinburgh: Elsevier.

References

Blumenthal, K.G., Peter, J.G., Trubiano, J.A. and Phillips, E.J. 2019. Antibiotic allergy. *Lancet*. **393**(10167), pp. 183–98.

BMJ 2017. Penicillin allergy: Getting the label right. *British Medical Journal* **358**, J3402. Available at www.bmj.com/content/358/bmj.j3402 (accessed 27 February 2023).

BNF 2023. *British National Formulary*. Available at bnf.nice.org.uk/ (accessed 27 February 2023).

BSAC 2018. *Antimicrobial Stewardship: From Principles to Practice*. British Society for Antimicrobial Chemotherapy. Available at bsac.org.uk/antimicrobial-stewardship-from-principles-to-practice-e-book/ (accessed 27 February 2023).

Burgess A. 2021. *How should Medicines be Dosed in Children who are Obese?* Specialist Pharmacy Service (SPS). Available at www.sps.nhs.uk/articles/how-should-medicines-be-dosed-in-children-who-are-obese/ (accessed 12 December 2022).

Cooke, J., Butler, C., Hopstaken, R., Dryden, M.S., McNulty, C., Hurding, S., Moore, M. and Livermore, D.M. 2015. Narrative review of primary care point-of-care testing (POCT) and antibacterial use in respiratory tract infection (RTI). *BMJ Open Respiratory Research.* **2**(1), pe000086.

Department of Health and Social Care (DHSC) 2019. *Tackling Antimicrobial Resistance 2019–2024: The UK's Five-year National Action Plan.* Global and Public Health Group, Emergency Preparedness and Health Protection Policy Directorate. Available at www.gov.uk/government/publications/uk-5-year-action-plan-for-antimicrobial-resistance-2019-to-2024 (accessed 18 April 2023).

Fulton, R.D.L. (chair), et al. 2005. *Guidelines on the Management of Cellulitis in Adults.* Northern Ireland: Clinical Resource Efficiency Support Team (CREST).

Garraghan, F. and Fallon, R. 2015. Gentamicin: Dose regimens and monitoring. *Pharmaceutical Journal.* **295**, pp. 7874–5.

Hand, K. and Joseph, A. 2021. *Clinical Breakpoints and Antimicrobial Dosing in Practice.* United Kingdom Clinical Pharmacist Association. Available at members. ukclinicalpharmacy.org/getattachment/Library/Webinars/PIN-Breakpoints-webinar-07-01-2021-slides.pdf.aspx?lang=en-GB (accessed 27 February 2023).

Ikuta, K.S., Swetschinski, L.R., Aguilar, G.R., Sharara, F., Mestrovic, T., Gray, A.P., Weaver, N.D., Wool, E.E., Han, C., Hayoon, A.G. and Aali, A., 2022. Global mortality associated with 33 bacterial pathogens in 2019: a systematic analysis for the Global Burden of Disease Study 2019. *The Lancet*, 400(10369), pp.2221-2248.

IIversen, K., Ihlemann, N., Gill, S.U., Madsen, T., Elming, H., Jensen, K.T., Bruun, N.E., Høfsten, D.E., Fursted, K., Christensen, J.J., Schultz, M., Klein, C.F., Fosbøll, E.L., Rosenvinge, F., Schønheyder, H.C., Køber, L. Torp-Pedersen, C., Helweg-Larsen, J., Tønder, N. et al. 2018. Partial oral versus intravenous antibiotic treatment of endocarditis. *New England Journal of Medicine.* **380**(5), pp. 415–24.

Leeds Teaching Hospitals NHS Trust (LTHT) 2023. *Blood Sciences Biochemistry and Haematology.* Available at www.leedsth.nhs.uk/a-z-of-services/pathology/blood-sciences/useful-information-and-links/ (accessed 27 February 2023).

Levine, A.R., Tran, M., Shepherd, J. and Naut, E. 2018. Utility of initial procalcitonin values to predict urinary tract infection. *American Journal of Emergency Medicine.* **36** (11), pp. 1993–7.

Li, H.-K., Rombach, I., Zambellas, R., Walker, A.S., McNally, M.A., Atkins, B.L., Lipsky, B.A., Hughes, H.C., Bose, D., Kümin, M., Scarborough, C., Matthews, P.C., Bfrent, A.J., Lomas, J., Gundle, R., Rogers, M., Taylor, A., Angus, B., Byren, I. et al. 2019. Oral versus intravenous antibiotics for bone and joint infection. *New England Journal of Medicine.*

380(5), pp. 425–36. Available at www.who.int/health-topics/infection-prevention-and-control#tab=tab_1 (accessed 18 November 2023).

Li, J.S., Sexton, D.J., Mick, N., Nettles, R., Fowler Jr, V.G., Ryan, T., Bashmore, T. and Corey, R. 2000. Proposed modifications to the Duke criteria for the diagnosis of infective endocarditis. *Clinical Infectious Diseases*. **30**(4), pp. 633–8.

Lim, W., Van der Eerden, M.M., Laing, R., Boersma, W.G., Karalus, N., Town, G.I., Lewis, S.A. and Macfarlane, J.T. 2003. Defining community acquired pneumonia severity on presentation to hospital: An international derivation and validation study. *Thorax*. **58**(8), pp. 377–82.

Llewelyn, M.J., Fitzpatrick, J.M., Darwin, E., Tonkin-Crine, S., Gorton, C., Paul, J., Peto, T.E.A., Yardley, L., Hopkins, S. and Walker, A.S. 2017. The antibiotic course has had its day. *British Medical Journal*. **358**(j3418).

Mantzourani, E., Cannings-John, R., Evans, A. and Ahmed, H. 2022. To swab or not to swab? Using point-of-care tests to detect Group A Streptococcus infections as part of a Sore Throat Test and Treat service in community pharmacy. *Journal of Antimicrobial Chemotherapy*. **77**(3), pp. 803–6.

Microbiology Society 2022. *The History of Antibiotics*. Available at microbiologysociety. org/members-outreach-resources/outreach-resources/antibiotics-unearthed/ antibiotics-and-antibiotic-resistance/the-history-of-antibiotics.html (accessed 30 August 2022).

Myo, J., Pooley, S. and Brennan, F. 2021. Oral, in place of intravenous, paracetamol as the new normal for elective cases. *Anaesthesia*. **76**(8), pp. 1143–4.

Nelson, R.E., Hatfiled, K.M., Wolford, H., Samore, M.H., Scott, R.D., Reddy, S.C., Olubajo, B., Paul, P., Jernigan, J.A. and Baggs, J. 2021. National estimates of healthcare costs associated with multidrug-resistant bacterial infections among hospitalized patients in the United States. *Clinical Infectious Diseases*. **72**(S1), pp. S17–S26.

NHS England 2019. *The NHS Long Term Plan*. Available at www.longtermplan.nhs.uk/ wp-content/uploads/2019/08/nhs-long-term-plan-version-1.2.pdf (accessed 31 May 2023).

NHS England 2021. *NHS Standard Contract 2021/22 Service Conditions (Full Length)*. Available at www.england.nhs.uk/publication/nhs-standard-contract-service-conditions-full-length/ (accessed 31 May 2023).

NHS England 2022. *Interactions: Antibiotics*. Available at www.nhs.uk/conditions/antibiotics/ interactions/ (accessed 18 April 2023).

NICE 2015a. *Antimicrobial Stewardship: Systems and Processes for Effective Antimicrobial Medicine Use*. Available at www.nice.org.uk/guidance/ng15 (accessed 8 January 2023).

NICE 2015b. *Sepsis: Recognition, Diagnosis and Early Management*. Available at www.nice.org. uk/guidance/ng51 (accessed 5 February 2023).

NICE 2018b. *Sore Throat (Acute) in Adults: Antimicrobial Prescribing*. Available at www.nice. org.uk/guidance/ng84/resources/sore-throat-acute-in-adults-antimicrobial-prescribing-pdf-1837694694085 (accessed 5 February 2023).

NICE 2018c. *Pyelonephritis (Acute): Antimicrobial Prescribing*. Available at www.nice.org.uk/ guidance/ng111/resources/pyelonephritis-acute-antimicrobial-prescribing-pdf-66141593379781 (accessed 27 February 2023).

NICE 2022a. *Antimicrobial Stewardship*. Available at www.nice.org.uk/guidance/health-protection/communicable-diseases/antimicrobial-stewardship (accessed 12 December 2022).

NICE 2022b. *Clinical Knowledge Summary: Diarrhoea – Antibiotic Associated*. Available at cks.nice.org.uk/topics/diarrhoea-antibiotic-associated/background-information/definition/ (accessed 6 November 2022).

NICE 2022c. *Clinical Knowledge Summary: Urinary Tract Infection (Lower) Women*. Available at cks.nice.org.uk/topics/urinary-tract-infection-lower-women/ (accessed 21 February 2022).

NICE 2022d. *Summary of Antimicrobial Prescribing Guidance: Managing Common Infections*. Available at www.bnf.org/news/2021/07/29/bnf-hosts-antimicrobial-summary-guidance-on-behalf-of-nice-and-phe/ (accessed 5 February 2023).

NIHR 2022. National Institute for Health Research *Double Check Patients with 'Penicillin Allergy' to Avoid Increased MRSA Risk*. Available at evidence.nihr.ac.uk/alert/are-you-sure-you-are-allergic-to-penicillin/ (accessed 31 May 2023).

Nogrady, B. 2016. *The Post-antibiotic Era will be a Frightening Place to Live: But There May be Ways to Avoid Disaster*. BBC. Available at www.bbc.com/future/article/20161010-all-you-need-to-know-about-the-antibiotic-apocalypse (accessed 31 May 2023).

Nuffield Trust 2021. *Antibiotic Prescribing*. Available at www.nuffieldtrust.org.uk/resource/antibiotic-prescribing (accessed on 8 December 2022).

Pfizer 2018. *Summary of Product Characteristics: Zyvox 600mg Film Coated Tablets*. Available at www.medicines.org.uk/emc/medicine/9857#gref (accessed 18 April 2023).

Pouwels, K.B., Hopkins, S., Llewelyn, M.J., Walker, A.S., McNulty, C.A.M. and Robotham, J.V. 2019. Duration of antibiotic treatment for common infections in English primary care: Cross sectional analysis and comparison with guidelines. *BMJ*. **364**, p. l440.

Public Health England (PHE) 2015. *Start Smart: Then Focus. Antimicrobial Stewardship Toolkit for English Hospitals*. Available at www.gov.uk/government/publications/antimicrobial-stewardship-start-smart-then-focus (accessed 31 May 2023).

Reygaert, W.C. 2018. An overview of the antimicrobial resistance mechanisms of bacteria. *AIMS Microbiology*. **4**(3), pp. 482–501.

Royal College of General Practitioners (RCGP) 2019. *TARGET: Treat Antibiotics Responsibly, Guidance, Education and Tools*. Available at elearning.rcgp.org.uk/course/view.php?id=553 (accessed 5 February 2023).

Royal College of Physicians (RCP) 2017. *National Early Warning Score (NEWS) 2: Standardising the Assessment of Acute-illness Severity in the NHS*. Available at www.rcplondon.ac.uk/projects/outputs/national-early-warning-score-news-2 (accessed 22 February 2023).

RPS 2021. *A Competency Framework for All Prescribers*. Available at www.rpharms.com/resources/frameworks/prescribing-competency-framework/competency-framework (accessed 12 May 2023).

Spinks, A., Glasziou, P.P. and Del Mar, C.B. 2021. Antibiotics for treatment of sore throat in children and adults. *Cochrane Database of Systematic Reviews*. **12**.

Strebhardt, K. and Ullrich, A. 2008. Paul Ehrlich's magic bullet concept: 100 years of progress. *Nature Reviews: Cancer*. **8**(6), pp. 473–80.

Stokes, M. and Abdijadid, S. 2022. *Disulfiram. StatPearls.* National Library of Medicine. Available at www.ncbi.nlm.nih.gov/books/NBK459340/ (accessed 18 April 2023).

United Kingdom Clinical Pharmacy Association (UKCPA) 2013. *Drug Dosing in Extremes of Body Weight in Critically Ill Patients.* 1st ed. Available at ukclinicalpharmacy.org/wp-content/uploads/2017/07/Drug-dosing-in-extremes-of-body-weight-2013.pdf (accessed 12 December 2022).

United Kingdom Health Security Agency (UKHSA) 2022. *AMR Local Indicators.* Available at fingertips.phe.org.uk/profile/amr-local-indicators (accessed 20 February 2023).

UKHSA 2023. *AMR Local Indicators.* Available at fingertips.phe.org.uk/profile/amr-local-indicators (accessed 20 February 2023).

UK Sepsis Trust 2022. *The Sepsis Manual.* 6th ed. Available at sepsistrust.org/professional-resources/education-resources/ (accessed 12 December 2022).

Waller, D.G. and Sampson, A.P. 2018. *Medical Pharmacology and Therapeutics.* 5th ed. Edinburgh: Elsevier.

World Health Organization (WHO) 2016. *Global Action Plan on Antimicrobial Resistance.* Available at www.who.int/publications/i/item/9789241509763 (accessed 18 April 2023).

WHO 2021a. *Antimicrobial Resistance.* Available at www.who.int/news-room/fact-sheets/detail/antimicrobial-resistance (accessed 31 January 2023).

WHO 2021b. *Infection Prevention and Control.* Available at www.who.int/teams/integrated-health-services/infection-prevention-control (accessed 31 May 2023).

7

Medicines Requiring Particular Care when Prescribing

Natalie Bryars

Chapter summary

This chapter discusses the risk in prescribing a number of specific drugs and drug groups. It identifies medicines which are most frequently cited as causing severe harm. In particular:

- oral methotrexate
- oral anticoagulants
- insulin
- opioids
- oral chemotherapy
- medicines for epilepsy.

Introduction

Care should be taken with all medicines to ensure that they are prescribed safely and effectively. However, some medicines require particular care as they are associated with a greater prevalence of prescribing errors or can cause significant harm when prescribed incorrectly.

In Competency 4, Prescribe, in the *RPS Competency Framework for All Prescribers* (RPS, 2021), there are two statements supporting the competency. These are: 4.1 'Prescribes a medicine or device with up-to-date awareness of its actions, indications, dose, contraindications, interactions, cautions and adverse effects' and 4.2 'Understands the potential for adverse effects and takes steps to recognise, and manage them, whilst minimising risk'.

In Competency 5, Provide information, there are two statements supporting the competency: 5.3 'Guides the patient/carer on how to identify reliable sources of information about their condition, medicines and treatment' and 5.5 'Encourages and supports the patient/carer to take responsibility for their medicines and self-manage their condition'.

Identifying medicines that are most frequently associated with severe harm

In 2001, the National Patient Safety Agency (NPSA) started to collect information on medication errors using the National Reporting and Learning System (NRLS). Through this, it identified the medicines most frequently associated with severe harm (Cousins et al., 2012). The top five were shown to be opioids, antibiotics, warfarin, low molecular weight heparin and insulin. With the potential dosing errors being an issue, methotrexate and oral anticancer drugs are included, as well as drugs for the treatment of epilepsy, with more recent warnings and advice. We have already covered antibiotics in Chapter 6.

Prior to 2012, when trends were identified, national patient safety alerts (NPSAs) were issued which contained recommendations to prevent recurrence. Healthcare organisations then had a responsibility to implement these and prevent patient harm. This has resulted in the creation of the category *never events*; organisations that have implemented safe processes should be able to prevent these errors and they should no longer happen. Any never event that does occur must be declared to NRLS and fully investigated using the serious incident framework.

In 2012, key functions and expertise for patient safety developed by the NPSA transferred to NHS England (www.england.nhs.uk/2012/05/npsa-transfer/), which works with NHS Improvement as a single organisation to improve patient care and provide leadership and support to the NHS. They continue to release NPSAs and annual summaries of incidents reported on NRLS, together with actions taken. These can be accessed at www.england.nhs.uk/patient-safety/patient-safety-alerts and help you to know the medicines that require particular care when you prescribe them and steps you can take to ensure patient safety. The never events policy, framework and list are reviewed regularly by NHS Improvement and can be accessed at www.england.nhs.uk/publication/never-events. NICE produces monthly medicines and prescribing support called 'Important new evidence', which includes any safety warnings from the Medicines and Healthcare products Regulatory Agency (MHRA) and manufacturers, and NPSAs. These can be accessed via the NICE website. You can also choose to have a monthly email with this information.

A note on NPSA alerts

On the website there are details about the earlier NPSA material. Alerts pre-2012 are now archived. The alerts and guidance that remain available on the archived NPSAs should be used with great caution.

Alerts have a distinctly different function to clinical guidelines and therefore are not routinely updated or reissued. When new, more effective interventions or resources to address a patient safety issue are identified, the potential to issue a new NPSA will be considered.

The archived early NPSA alerts can be found at webarchive.nationalarchives.gov.uk/ukgwa/20171030124143/http://www.nrls.npsa.nhs.uk/resources/type/alerts/

Oral methotrexate

Methotrexate is used to treat a number of non-cancer indications, such as rheumatoid arthritis, psoriasis and Crohn's disease (not licensed for use in severe Crohn's disease). In these cases, it is prescribed as a once-weekly dose. However, dosing errors were a common cause of severe patient harm, especially when methotrexate was prescribed more frequently than once weekly. This led to a patient safety alert being issued to improve compliance with oral methotrexate guidelines. This has been so well publicised by the NPSA that NHS Improvement (2018) has classed methotrexate being prescribed more frequently than once weekly for these patients as a 'never event'. This means that the error is entirely preventable and should never happen. However, a considerable number of reports of serious toxicity due to inadvertent daily dosing led to additional prescribing advice being issued (MHRA, 2020). In the BNF, the MHRA 'Important safety information' is given to emphasise safe methotrexate prescribing.

When prescribing oral methotrexate, you should always include the correct:

- dose
- route
- frequency
- day of the week when methotrexate should be taken.

Whenever you prescribe methotrexate, you should make sure you are informing patients or their carers about how to take methotrexate safely and that they are able to comply with once-weekly dosing. A patient reminder card is available to help with this (gov.uk, 2020), together with educational materials for healthcare professionals. This includes information about potential side-effects and how these should be managed to reduce the risk of patient harm. In addition, what other medicines the patient is taking should be considered; only one strength of methotrexate tablet should be used for patients on oral dosing, usually 2.5mg tablets. In the *Competency Framework for All Prescribers* (RPS, 2021), Competency 5, Provide information, includes five supporting statements each linked to this requirement.

Methotrexate is a cytotoxic drug and every patient who takes it needs to be closely monitored. Serious patient harm can occur if the correct monitoring is not conducted.

Question 7.1

What monitoring do you think needs to take place when methotrexate is prescribed for non-cancer indications?

Answer 7.1

For all patients prescribed methotrexate, the full blood count, liver function tests and renal function tests need to be closely reviewed. Patients also need to be monitored for signs of methotrexate toxicity/intolerance, such as breathlessness, dry persistent cough, vomiting, diarrhoea, sore throat, bruising or mouth ulcers.

Methotrexate affects folate metabolism and can cause side-effects that are similar to folate deficiency. Patients who experience mucosal or gastrointestinal side-effects may benefit from folic acid. Although this is an unlicensed indication, as long as it is not taken on the same day as methotrexate, the effectiveness of methotrexate has not been shown to be reduced. In the monograph for methotrexate, in the BNF, as well as the MHRA safety information, there is a section 'Cautions: Further information' which you should read. It covers such things as potential liver, gastric and cardiac toxicity as well as bone marrow suppression (BNF, 2022).

Anticoagulants

Anticoagulants are a class of medicines that are commonly identified as causing patient harm and hospital admissions (Pirmohamed et al., 2004). The NPSA undertook a literature review and completed a risk assessment on the use of anticoagulants in the NHS. This found that inadequate competencies of healthcare professionals prescribing and monitoring patients on anticoagulants and failure to implement professional guidelines contributed to the high incidence of patient harm.

The BNF has sections on both oral and parenteral anticoagulants which you should read if this is an area you are likely to be involved in.

Do you have the knowledge and training needed to prescribe anticoagulants safely? E-learning packages are available to assist with the initiation and maintenance of anticoagulant therapy at: learning.bmj.com/learning/; type anticoagulation in the search box. Additional e-learning packages for anticoagulant therapy are available at: www.e-lfh.org.uk/safe-prescribing-foundation-elearning-programme-update-august-2022/safe anticoagulation

Oral anticoagulants

The BNF section on oral anticoagulants explains the main use of the drugs and the use of the International Normalised Ratio (INR) in various conditions.

Warfarin

Warfarin is currently the most commonly prescribed anticoagulant (www.nhs.uk/conditions/anticoagulants, updated 2021). It can be difficult to prescribe as dosing is specific to each individual patient. Over-anticoagulation can cause patient harm through haemorrhage and under-anticoagulation can cause patient harm through thrombosis, both of which can be life threatening.

The British Society for Haematology has produced clear guidelines for the management of patients taking warfarin (Keeling et al., 2011). These are reviewed regularly and, when appropriate, updated.

Activity 7.2

Read Keeling et al., 2011 (see References; available at b-s-h.org.uk/guidelines/?search=warfarin).

What are the key learning points for you as a future prescriber of anticoagulants?

Answer 7.2

Before you initiate a patient on warfarin, you should be clear about:

- the indication;
- the target INR;
- the duration of treatment;
- if the patient is at high risk from warfarinisation (e.g., has congestive cardiac failure, infection, interacting drugs, liver failure, diarrhoea, a raised baseline INR);
- if the patient has any contraindications;
- the loading regime (an age-related dosing algorithm should always be followed when fast-loading of warfarin is required);
- if parenteral anticoagulation is required until oral anticoagulation with warfarin is established;
- if the patient is of childbearing potential (warfarin is teratogenic and should not be given in the first trimester of pregnancy. It can also increase risk of haemorrhage and should be avoided in the last trimester of pregnancy).

You need to carry out or order baseline tests before warfarin therapy can be started. These include a baseline INR, LFTs, activated partial thromboplastin time (APPT) and platelets. Are you confident about how to interpret each of these tests? Additional information can be found at labtestsonline.org.uk/tests-index

You also need to be confident that the patient is fully able to manage their warfarin therapy, as well as being able to attend frequent INR monitoring – something especially important in patients that are frail, confused, or who have chaotic lifestyles (Keeling et al., 2011).

You need to give appropriate counselling to all patients and/or their carers who are prescribed oral anticoagulants at the start of their therapy. The *Competency Framework for All Prescribers* (RPS, 2021) includes discussions and consultations with patients and carers in a number of the competencies. For example, in Competency 5, Providing information, supporting statement 5.2 states: 'Checks the patient's/carer's understanding of the discussions had, actions needed and their commitment to the management plan'. There are many others in other competencies which you should look at.

Booklets are available, which provide patients with essential information about warfarin, including potential side-effects and how they should be managed. The booklets also have sections for recording details about the patient's dose and blood test results and a card for the patient's purse or wallet, which alerts others to the fact that they are taking warfarin. Booklets can be obtained from www.medicines.org.uk/emc/rmm/1081/Document

Be clear about who will be responsible for dosing the patient and monitoring them. Most patients are managed by an anticoagulant service. If you make a referral to an anticoagulant service, you need to make sure that you provide them with all the information they need to dose the patient effectively. This includes the diagnosis, the target INR, the planned duration of treatment, the dose of warfarin on referral and any current medication (Keeling et al., 2011).

Monitoring warfarin

Warfarin interacts with a wide range of medications (see BNF, appendix 1, or interactions on the NICE-BNF website), many producing an increase in anticoagulant effect. It can also be affected by changes in diet and alcohol consumption. As a prescriber, you should be aware of this and make appropriate prescribing decisions and dose adjustments. Many fatalities and permanent harm events with warfarin were associated with inadequate laboratory monitoring and clinically significant drug interactions, usually involving non-steroidal anti-inflammatories such as ibuprofen or diclofenac.

Direct-acting oral anticoagulants

A range of direct-acting oral anticoagulants (DOACs) are available, including apixaban, dabigatran, edoxaban and rivaroxaban, and their use is becoming increasingly common. They are licensed for a range of therapeutic indications and do not require regular blood tests for monitoring the INR. Instead, dosage is determined by indication, age, body weight, renal function, drug interactions and patient factors. However, they are not suitable for all patients. See the BNF for licensed indications and prescribing information or the EMC at www.medicines.org.uk/emc for each of the drugs mentioned.

Parenteral anticoagulants

Again, the BNF has a section on parenteral anticoagulants which you should read. It mentions heparin and low molecular weight heparins. Heparin is an injectable anticoagulant. It is used in higher doses to treat venous and arterial thromboembolism, as well as in lower doses for thromboprophylaxis. It is fast-acting, so is often used until oral anticoagulation can be established, as well as at times when oral anticoagulants are deemed unsuitable. Heparins have a section on their own in the BNF which also has a section on unfractionated heparins. If checking the index, you need to look up heparins, unfractionated.

Unfractionated heparins

Therapeutic doses of sodium and calcium heparin have to be monitored on a regular basis. This ensures that the dose being given is achieving the required level of anticoagulation and the most common way to test this is with the APPT test.

Both inadequate laboratory monitoring and inappropriate dosing can cause harm to patients in secondary care. This is because frequent dose adjustments are usually required to ensure effective anticoagulation and to minimise the risk of bleeding through excessive anticoagulation.

Low molecular weight heparins

These are found (under this name) in the BNF. Low molecular weight heparins (LMWHs) are manufactured from unfractionated heparins. They have a lower molecular weight, which gives them different anticoagulant and pharmacokinetic properties to unfractionated heparins. They are used both to treat venous and arterial thromboembolism and for thromboprophylaxis in the majority of hospitals within the UK. Low molecular weight heparins are prescribed according to the weight of the patient for many indications and blood tests are not generally needed to ensure effective anticoagulation.

Frequent causes of patient harm include failure to weigh patients accurately, failure to identify the clinical need to initiate treatment and an inability to calculate an appropriate dose. The renal function of the patient also needs to be taken into consideration. LMWH is renally cleared and must be used with caution in patients with renal failure due to an increased risk of bleeding. In these patients, you may need to reduce the dose or use an unfractionated heparin. You can find further dosing information in the BNF.

Activity 7.3

Look at a current copy of the BNF, use the app or go online and read about the low molecular weight heparins currently licensed for use. What dose of dalteparin would you prescribe for a female patient with deep vein thrombosis who has normal renal function and weighs 62kg?

Answer 7.3

Dalteparin 12,500 units should be prescribed once daily by subcutaneous injection until adequate anticoagulation with a vitamin K antagonist, such as warfarin, is established (at least five days of combined treatment is usually required). A dose of 200 units per kilogram daily is indicated giving a dose of 12,400 units. However, dalteparin is available as a pre-filled syringe and dose banding is used to determine the most appropriate syringe, which in this case is 12,500 units.

Insulin

Between November 2003 and November 2009 there were a high number of reports of medication incidents involving insulin. Common causes of patient harm included:

- inappropriate doses being prescribed or administered;
- the wrong type of insulin being prescribed or administered;
- inappropriate abbreviation of the term 'unit' leading to ten-times dose administration errors;
- delayed or omitted doses.

Look at the chapter on insulins in the BNF. You will see that there are over 30 different types of insulin available in the UK at present. They can be human insulin analogues or extracted from animals. They can be rapid-acting, intermediate-acting or long-acting. They are available as a mixture of different insulins, known as biphasic insulins. They are also available in a number of different injection formats. Can you see the potential for confusion when prescribing or administering insulin especially with insulins that have similar sounding names, such as Novorapid and Novomix; or insulins that have small differences in their descriptors, such as Humalog, Humalog Mix25 and Humalog Mix50; or insulins that are available in different strengths?

Always prescribe insulins using the brand name. This should be written in full and the device specified. The type of insulin and strength should be recorded. The dose should also be written clearly and the word 'units' written in full.

Inappropriate dosing with insulin can cause severe patient harm and patient death. This has been so well publicised that NHS Improvement (2018) has classed it as a 'never event' if a patient is given an overdose due to an incorrect device being used or if a ten-fold or greater overdose is given because of the abbreviation of the words 'unit' or 'international units'.

Insulin syringes should always be used to measure and administer insulin from vials. Insulin must never be withdrawn from an insulin pen or pen refill and administered via a syringe. This, and other important safety information, is shown at the beginning of the 'Insulins' section of the BNF as a NHS Improvement Patient Safety Alert from 2016. The NHS 'never event' of overdose of insulin due to abbreviations or incorrect device is included from 2018 (BNF 84). Also in the section on Insulin in the BNF is MHRA advice about the injection site which you should read.

Activity 7.4

Look at the Insulins section in the BNF (online or hard copy) and read the various warnings and advice. The section then divides up into three different insulin types. Identify these ?

Answer 7.4

Insulins

Short acting (includes soluble insulin and Rapid-acting insulin)

Intermediate-acting

Long-acting

There are also insulins combined with other glucose-lowering medicines such as liraglutide and lixisenatide.

In each main section there are many individual medicinal forms which may have variations in licensing.

Do you know when, during the day, different insulins should be prescribed for administration? Rapid-acting insulin analogues are usually given with or immediately after meals. Short-acting insulins are usually given 15–30 minutes before meals and in diabetic emergencies. Biphasic insulins are a mix of a rapid-acting and an intermediate-acting insulin and are usually given two or three times a day with meals. Intermediate- and long-acting insulins are usually given once or twice a day.

Do you have the knowledge and training needed to prescribe insulin safely? E-learning packages are available to assist with the prescribing and administration of insulin. The training package 'Six steps to insulin safety' is endorsed by Diabetes UK and is available at www.diabetes.org.uk. The BNF will also provide you with essential prescribing information about different insulins. In addition, MIMS (Monthly Index of Medical Specialities) online will give you information about administration and the duration of action of each insulin (www.mims.co.uk). Guidance on prescribing insulin in type 1 diabetes (NICE, 2015) and type 2 diabetes (NICE, 2017) is also available.

Activity 7.5

Complete the e-learning package on the safe use of insulin from NHS Diabetes at www.diabetes.org.uk/professionals/training–competencies/courses#E-learning or diabetesonthenet.com/cpd-modules/the-six-steps-to-insulin-safety/ What are the key learning points for you as a future prescriber of insulin?

Patients should also be empowered to take an active role in their treatment with insulin. In support of this, the insulin passport was developed by NHS Diabetes and supported by Diabetes UK. This documents the patient's current insulin regime and enables a safety check for you as the prescriber. Prescribers are required to provide insulin passports when initiating or providing repeat prescriptions for insulin and local versions can be obtained from GP surgeries, specialist nurses and diabetes centres. In addition, a patient information leaflet describing the safe use of insulin is available at www.england.nhs.uk/improvement-hub/wp-content/uploads/sites/44/2017/11/Safe-use-of-insulin-and-you-patient-info-booklet.pdf

Opioids

Opioids are commonly used to treat acute and chronic pain. However, the NPSA received a high number of dose-related patient safety incidents concerning opioids, mainly due to inappropriate doses being prescribed or administered. This was especially true when the patient had no history of taking opioids and could be very sensitive to their effects.

Whenever you prescribe an opioid, you must take a full patient history to determine any previous opioid use. This includes the doses, formulations and the frequencies of both regular and as required opioids. This enables you to make sure that the dose you are prescribing is safe for the patient.

Information on starting doses, as well as dose conversions, of opioids is available in the BNF and can be found under each individual drug name, or in the 'Prescribing in palliative care' section at the beginning of the formulary. Additional information can also be sourced in the *Palliative Care Formulary* (Twycross et al., 2006), in local policies and guidelines or, alternatively, go to www.medicinescomplete.com. This is an online platform providing access to a range of drug and healthcare resources that is accessible to most people working in the NHS.

When you increase the dose of an opioid, you should make sure that the calculated dose is safe for the patient. Dose increases should not normally be more than 30–50 per cent higher than the previous dose.

Wrong product selection is another common cause of errors. You should therefore make sure you are familiar with all the products you are prescribing.

Activity 7.6

Do you know the difference between these products?

Oxycodone 10mg modified-release tablets

Oxycodone 10mg capsules

Oxycodone oral solution 1mg in 1mL

Answer 7.6

Oxycodone modified-release tablets should be prescribed twice daily and doses administered at 12-hour intervals.

Oxycodone is twice as potent as morphine.

Oxycodone capsules or oral liquid are immediate-release preparations and should be prescribed for acute pain relief and breakthrough pain.

Case 7.1

A palliative patient with chronic pain has been well controlled on oral morphine, taking morphine sulphate modified-release tablets (MST) 30mg twice daily for several months. They have compliance problems due to difficulties in swallowing tablets and a decision is made to start them on fentanyl patches. What dose of patch would you prescribe for them? How should they apply it? When would you advise them to stop taking their MST and start with the fentanyl patches? What would you prescribe them for breakthrough analgesia?

Response 7.1

Review the palliative care section in the BNF or the SmPC on www.medicines.org.uk for fentanyl patches to determine equivalent doses of opioid analgesics. A fentanyl 25 microgram per hour patch is equivalent to 60mg of oral morphine in 24 hours.

Review the fentanyl directions for administration section in the BNF. One patch should be applied to dry, non-hairy, non-irradiated skin on the upper arm or torso. It should be removed every 72 hours and replaced with a new patch, sited on a different area. The patient should also avoid exposure of patches to heat, including hot water.

Review the SmPC. Evaluation of the analgesic effect should not be undertaken until the patch has been in place for at least 24 hours as it takes time to achieve steady-state concentrations. The previous analgesia should be phased out gradually, with the last dose of MST being taken at the time the first patch is applied.

Review the prescribing in palliative care section in the BNF. If pain occurs, immediate-release morphine can be prescribed for breakthrough pain, such as morphine sulphate oral solution if the patient can swallow liquids. The dose is usually one-tenth to one-sixth of the regular total daily dose, given every two to four hours if necessary. Formulations of fentanyl that are given via the nasal, buccal or sublingual route are also licensed for breakthrough pain. The number of doses taken for breakthrough pain and the patient's response to them should be monitored and considered when making dose adjustments to the fentanyl patch.

See the section on controlled drugs in Chapter 10.

Guidance is available on the prescribing of controlled drugs, including making and recording prescribing decisions and providing information to patients or carers (NICE, 2016). The Misuse of Drugs Act (2001) means that there are many legal requirements relating to the prescribing of opioid analgesics. There is also a section in this book that discusses prescribing in general and prescribing of controlled drugs in particular (Chapter 10).

Oral anticancer medicines (chemotherapy)

Oral anticancer medicines are commonly administered in primary and secondary care. The NPSA received high numbers of patient safety incidents concerning oral anticancer medication. This was reiterated by the MHRA in 2014 (www.gov.uk/drug-safety-update/oral-anticancer-medicines-risk-of-incorrect-dosing). Common causes of patient harm included:

- wrong doses being prescribed;
- wrong frequency being prescribed;
- wrong course duration being prescribed.

The standards for prescribing oral anticancer medicines should be the same as those for injectable chemotherapy. This means that they should only be initiated by a cancer specialist and prescribed only in the context of a written protocol or treatment plan. The patient should also be given full verbal and written confirmation about their oral cancer medication upon initiation. This must include details on the intended regime, the treatment plan and any monitoring arrangements that are in place.

If you are a non-cancer specialist, you may occasionally be asked to prescribe ongoing anticancer medication for a patient. In this case, discuss this with the cancer specialist first to ensure it is appropriate. However, if you are the specialist nurse your expertise will be needed.

In the *Competency Framework for All Prescribers*, Competency 10 is Prescribe as part of a team. This means you may be working with junior nurses and doctors and your expertise may be required. Supporting statement 10.4 states: 'Provides support and advice to other prescribers or those involved in administration of medicines where appropriate'. Make sure you have access to all written protocols and treatment plans, including guidance on monitoring and the management of toxicity, before you prescribe anything.

If you need them, your local cancer alliance can provide you with a range of chemotherapy education resources. They can also provide you with the local treatment protocols and relevant patient information. If you do not know how to access your local cancer alliance, log on to www.england.nhs.uk/cancer/cancer-alliances and you will be directed.

Antiepileptic medicines

A large number of medicines are used in the management of epilepsy. These can be reviewed in the BNF in the section on epilepsy and other seizures. Different antiepileptic medicines have different properties but all are used for the purpose of controlling epilepsy by preventing seizures. Guidance on prescribing antiepileptic medicines is available to you (NICE, 2022). This covers the diagnosis of epilepsy, support and information for patients, treatment of epilepsy, monitoring of treatment and treatment withdrawal. The choice of treatment depends on the presenting epilepsy syndrome, seizure type and a wide range of patient factors. Medication regimes therefore need to be individualised and finely titrated to be effective.

Generic and brand prescribing of antiepileptic medicines

Many antiepileptic medicines are available in both generic and branded forms. These can vary in characteristics, meaning that there can be risks to patients when switching them between products made by different manufacturers. In Chapter 10 we discuss generic and brand prescribing generally. It is important that you are aware of this as changing or not specifying the brand on an antiepileptic prescription could harm the patient, causing adverse effects or a reduction in seizure control. To help you with this, guidance has been issued on switching between different manufacturers' products for antiepileptic medicines (MHRA, 2017). This states that antiepileptic medicines can be classified into three categories based on therapeutic index, solubility and absorption. For each category, advice is available on the necessity of continuing the supply of a specific manufacturer's product for use in epilepsy. These are also listed in the BNF (2022; see, specifically, bnf.nice.org.uk/treatment-summaries/epilepsy/).

For example, in Category 1 you should ensure that patients are maintained on the specific manufacturer's antiepileptic medicines which include carbamazepine and phenytoin.

In Category 2 you, as the prescriber, must use your clinical judgement on the need to maintain the specific manufacturer's preparation. Examples given are clonazepam and lamotrigine.

Finally, for preparations in Category 3 there should not usually be the need to maintain the specific manufacturer's product. For example, pregabalin and gabapentin.

Look at the BNF section which shows the three categories; familiarise yourself with the differences, particularly those preparations that are in Category 1 and should be maintained on the specific manufacturer's preparation.

If a specific manufacturer's product is required, this should be clearly written on the prescription by specifying a brand name or by using the generic name and name of the manufacturer.

Sodium Valproate

One antiepileptic medicine, valproate, is highly teratogenic and its use in pregnancy is associated with neurodevelopmental disorders and congenital malformations. This is such a high risk that guidance has been issued on prescribing valproate to female patients (MHRA, 2018). This states that valproate must not be prescribed for women and girls of childbearing potential unless certain requirements are met. These are as follows:

- the patient has been fully informed of the risks;
- a pregnancy prevention programme is in place;
- a risk acknowledgement form has been completed and signed;
- the risk acknowledgement form has been reviewed annually;
- no other effective treatments are available for the patient.

Supportive materials are available to help with this, including a patient booklet, a patient card, a booklet for healthcare professionals and an annual risk acknowledgement form. These can be downloaded from www.gov.uk/guidance/valproate-use-by-women-and-girls

From January 2024 new regulatory measures related to sodium valproate have been introduced by the MHRA, however the current safety measures continue to apply (MHRA, 2013).

Summary

Although care should be taken with all medicines to ensure that they are prescribed safely and effectively, some medicines require particular care as they are associated with a greater prevalence of prescribing errors or can cause significant harm when prescribed incorrectly. This chapter discussed the work of the NPSA, the key functions of which transferred to NHS England in 2012, and identified six specific medicines or medicine groups where extra care is essential. These were oral methotrexate, oral anticoagulants, insulin, opioids, oral chemotherapy and medicines for epilepsy.

References

Baglin, T., Barrowcliffe, W., Cohen, A. and Greaves, M. 2006. Guidelines on the use and monitoring of heparin. *British Journal of Haematology*. **133**, pp. 19–34.

BNF 2022. *British National Formulary: Key Information on the Selection, Prescribing, Dispensing and Administration of Medicines*. Available at bnf.nice.org.uk/ (accessed December 2022).

Cousins, D., Gerrett, D. and Warner, B. 2012. A review of medication incidents reported to the National Reporting and Learning System in England and Wales over 6 years (2005–2010). *British Journal of Clinical Pharmacology*. **74**(4), pp. 597–604.

gov.uk 2020. Methotrexate once-weekly for autoimmune diseases: new measures to reduce risk of fatal overdose due to inadvertent daily instead of weekly dosing. *Drug Safety Update*. Available at www.gov.uk/drug-safety-update/methotrexate-once-weekly-for-autoimmune-diseases-new-measures-to-reduce-risk-of-fatal-overdose-due-to-inadvertent-daily-instead-of-weekly-dosing (accessed 15 September 2023).

Keeling, D., Baglin, T., Tait, C., Watson, H., Perry, D., Baglin, C., Kitchen, S. and Makris, M. 2011. Guidelines on oral anticoagulation with warfarin fourth edition *British Journal of Haematology*. **154**(3), pp. 311–24.

Medicines and Healthcare products Regulatory Agency (MHRA) 2017. Antiepileptic Drugs: Updated Advice on Switching Between Different Manufacturers' Products. Available at www.gov.uk/drug-safety-update/antiepileptic-drugs-updated-advice-on-switching-between-different-manufacturers-products (accessed 15 September 2023).

MHRA 2013. Valproate: review of safety data and expert advice on management of risks Public Assessment Report. https://assets.publishing.service.gov.uk/media/65660310312f400013e5d508/Valproate-report-review-and-expert-advice.pdf

MHRA 2018. *Valproate Use by Women and Girls*. Available at www.gov.uk/guidance/valproate-use-by-women-and-girls (accessed 15 September 2023).

MHRA 2020. Methotrexate Once Weekly for Autoimmune Diseases: New Measures to Reduce Risk of Fatal Overdose Due to Inadvertent Daily Instead of Weekly Dosing. Available at www.gov.uk/drug-safety-update/methotrexate-once-weekly-for-autoimmune-diseases-new-measures-to-reduce-risk-of-fatal-overdose-due-to-inadvertent-daily-instead-of-weekly-dosing (accessed 15 September 2023).

Misuse of Drugs Regulations 2001. No 3998. Available at www.legislation.gov.uk/uksi/2001/3998/contents (accessed 15 September 2023).

NHS Improvement 2018. *The 'Never Events' List 2018 (last updated February 2021) CG 20/18*. Available at www.england.nhs.uk/publication/never-events/ (accessed 15 September 2023).

NICE 2015. *Type 1 Diabetes in Adults: Diagnosis and Management*. NG17. Available at www.nice.org.uk/guidance/ng17 (accessed December 2022).

NICE 2016. *Controlled Drugs: Safe Use and Management*. NG46. Available at www.nice.org.uk/guidance/ng46 (accessed December 2022).

NICE 2017. *Type 2 Diabetes in Adults: Management*. NG28. Available at www.nice.org.uk/guidance/ng28 (accessed December 2022).

NICE 2020. *Clinical Guide for the Management of Anticoagulant Services During the Coronavirus Pandemic*. 001559. Available at www.nice.org.uk www.nice.org.uk/media/default/about/covid-19/specialty-guides/specialty-guide-anticoagulant-services-and-coronavirus.pdf (accessed 15 September 2023).

NICE 2022. *Epilepsies in Children, Young People and Adults*. NG217. Available at www.nice.org.uk/guidance/ng217 (accessed December 2022).

Pirmohamed, M., James, S., Meakin, S., Green, C., Scott, A.K., Walley, T.J., Farrar, K., Park, B.K. and Breckenridge, A.M. 2004. Adverse drug reactions as a cause of admission to hospital: Prospective analysis of 18,820 patients. *BMJ*. **329**, pp. 15–19.

RPS 2021. *A Competency Framework for All Prescribers*. Available at www.rpharms.com/resources/frameworks/prescribing-competency-framework/competency-framework (accessed 12 May 2023).

Twycross, R., Wilcock, A., Charlesworth, S. and Dickman, A. 2006. *Palliative Care Formulary*. 2nd ed. Oxford: Radcliffe.

8

Prescribing for Particular Patient Groups

Daniel Greer

Chapter summary

The chapter explores the care needed when prescribing medicines in particular patient groups. Those selected in this chapter are:

- children
- patients with hepatic impairment
- patients with renal impairment
- pregnant women
- breast-feeding women
- older people.

Introduction

Within the *Competency Framework for All Prescribers* (RPS, 2021), Competency 2 is entitled Identifying evidence-based treatment options available for clinical decision making.

Supporting statements within this competency include 2.4, which takes into account how individual patient factors such as genetics, age, renal impairment and pregnancy affect pharmacokinetics and pharmacodynamics and how other patient factors such as ability to swallow, disability and visual impairment affect medicines choice, formulation and route.

There are many sources of information specific to the groups mentioned but the most important at this stage are the *British National Formulary* (BNF) and the *British National Formulary for Children* (BNFC) (see Chapter 2 for more detail). You can access these as a hard copy, via an app or online at bnf.nice.org.uk/

There are pages at the beginning of the BNF called 'Guidance on prescribing' which discuss prescribing in specific patient groups. As you would anticipate, the BNFC has more detail about prescribing for children – for example, how to administer medicines, oral syringes and managing medicines in school. Both the BNF and the BNFC should be consulted as you read this chapter and should be used as reference tools in future. If using the hard copies, ensure you are using the most up-to-date edition.

The list in **Box 8.1** gives the groups specifically selected for further discussion here and in the BNF 'Guidance on prescribing' section.

Box 8.1 Patient groups requiring greater care when prescribing

- Children
- Patients with hepatic impairment
- Patients with renal impairment
- Pregnant women
- Breast-feeding women
- Older people

You should take particular care when you are prescribing for patients in these groups as changes in pharmacokinetics and pharmacodynamics (see Chapter 6) mean that the potential for adverse drug reactions and prescribing errors may be higher among these patients. This chapter will explain the underlying factors that affect prescribing and give advice on principles to be followed and sources of information, in addition to the BNF and BNFC, that are best used to guide the choice of drugs and doses.

The selection of these groups and the order in which they are described is simply to mirror the BNF.

Prescribing for children

First, what do we mean by children? The BNFC has a table showing the definitions for different age groups. For example, a neonate is defined as from 0 up to 28 days or the first four weeks of life; an infant is from 28 days of life to 24 months; and a child is defined as being from two years to 12 years of age. Children are not simply small adults; they may differ from adults in their response to drugs and the way in which they handle them. The choice of dose is very important as there are huge variations in weight across the age range of birth to 18 years, and also large changes in physical development, which affect drug distribution, excretion and metabolism. The most dramatic changes occur in the first year of life (see also Batchelor and Marriott, 2015). Before we begin, look at the different doses of amoxicillin for different ages in the BNFC.

Activity 8.1

Look up the dose of amoxicillin for susceptible infections in the BNFC for:

- a neonate up to seven days;
- a neonate between seven to 28 days;
- child one to 11 months;
- a child one to four years;
- a child five to 11 years.

Answer 8.1

For susceptible infections:

Amoxicillin by IV infusion

A neonate up to seven days old by IV infusion 30mg/kg every 12 hours, increased if necessary to 60mg every 12 hours – used in severe infections.

By mouth

Neonate between seven and 28 days 30mg/kg three times a day, max per dose 125mg.

Child one to 11 months 125mg three times a day, increased if necessary up to 30mg/kg three times a day.

Child one to four years old 250mg three times a day, increased if necessary up to 30mg/kg three times a day.

Child five to 11 years old 500mg three times a day, increased if necessary to 1g three times a day. Use increased dose for severe infections.

This shows the importance of using the BNFC for child doses, particularly for neonates. The BNF does have some child doses for amoxicillin but only from one month of age, where they are the same as the BNFC. As mentioned, children are not simply small adults; great care is needed when deciding on the dose to give. Medication errors can lead to an increase in risk in paediatrics. Consequences of such errors can be significant. Most common errors are calculation-related so great care is needed when calculating doses. If you don't feel confident, check with a colleague.

There are important pharmacokinetic changes that occur in children.

Absorption

Gastric emptying in infants up to six months of age takes longer than in adults and may result in a slower rate of absorption; therefore onset of action may be delayed in neonates and young infants. Overall bioavailability (the proportion of a dose reaching the systemic circulation) generally remains the same, although it can be unpredictable.

You may be surprised to know that an increased topical absorption may be seen in neonates and infants due to the stratum corneum being thinner. As the body surface area to weight ratio is higher in this age group there is a greater potential for adverse effects. This may be especially relevant with topical steroids in children with eczema where the inflamed skin can further increase absorption.

You should generally avoid giving intramuscular injections in children. The lack of muscle mass means that injections can be very painful, and the variability in blood flow means that absorption into the systemic circulation can be unpredictable.

Distribution

Important changes in body fat/water composition occur in the first year. Fat content rises from 12 per cent to 30 per cent from term to one year, while body water drops from 75 per cent to 60 per cent. For water-soluble drugs, larger doses on a mg/kg basis may be required in a neonate compared to an older child in order to achieve therapeutic levels. Highly protein-bound drugs may also have altered distribution in neonates and infants as they generally have lower albumin concentrations and their foetal albumin is less efficient at binding drugs. This is likely to result in higher amounts of 'free' drug and potentially an increase in side-effects. See Chapter 6 for more about protein binding.

Metabolism

As we have already stated in Chapter 6, the liver is the main, though not only, site of metabolism of drugs. However, the liver may take up to two years after birth to reach full maturity for some enzyme pathways; thus drug metabolism is generally reduced in neonates and young children and doses may need to be reduced. From years one to five, however, metabolic activity increases compared to adults, and larger doses of hepatically metabolised drugs such as theophylline may be required compared to adults on a mg/kg basis.

Excretion

Renal function in neonates is less than adults; however, it undergoes rapid maturation during the first weeks post-birth in both term and preterm infants, before declining with age. Many drugs such as cephalosporins and penicillins or beta blockers are renally excreted so particular care is needed when prescribing them for the very young.

There are also some recognised differences in pharmacodynamics of medicines in children, with different types of adverse effects seen – for example, sodium valproate is more likely to cause hepatotoxicity in children under ten years than in adults; oculogyric crises with metoclopramide are more common in girls under 16 years than in adults. There are also data to show that for some drugs the blood levels needed for a particular effect are different to adults.

Sources of information on dosing

It is important to note that medication errors can be particularly serious in children and the most common errors are calculation-related. If you are regularly working with children as a prescriber, you should obtain a source of child doses of medicines from a paediatric and neonatal dosage handbook. The recommended gold standard source is the current edition of the BNFC in the UK, although the adult BNF contains some paediatric doses. There is also a very useful website called *Medicines for Children* which can be accessed at www.medicinesforchildren.org.uk/ and can be used by parents as well as you as the prescriber.

How do you calculate doses in paediatrics?

There are three main methods that you will come across when calculating doses for children.

Body weight

This is the most common method to calculate doses. In the BNFC, this is stated as a dose in milligrams per kilogram (mg/kg). Although not done as often as it might be, it is good practice to document body weight on prescriptions to allow doses to be double checked.

Body surface area

The use of body surface area (BSA) allows for comparison of results in children of various size and body composition. In addition, the dosing of some drugs such as cytotoxics and radio contrast drugs for imaging are based on BSA rather than weight alone. BSA can be calculated from weight using 'nomograms'. A table of BSA according to body weight is available at the back of the BNFC. Height is not required using those tables. If you have a hard copy BNFC, have look at it now or go online or use the app see how easy it is to find the BSA tables.

Dosing by age

Some drugs with a wide therapeutic range (see Chapter 6) are quoted as a single dose for an age range. However, you should take care if children are underweight for their age as this could result in an overdose. Tables of mean weight by age are available at the back of the BNFC.

Whatever method is used to calculate the dose, make sure that the dose can be practically measured. An oral syringe should be used for accurate measurement and controlled administration of oral liquid medicine. The standard oral syringe is supplied when liquid medicines are prescribed in doses other than multiples of 5mL and is marked in 0.5mL divisions (1mL syringes are also available with 0.1mL divisions). The BNFC discusses administration of medicine to children under the section 'Guidance on prescribing'.

Dose frequency

Antibacterials are generally given at regular intervals throughout the day. Some flexibility should be allowed in children to avoid waking them during the night. For example, the night-time dose may be given at the child's bedtime. It is also good practice to avoid administration during the school day if at all possible – for example, consider whether the lunchtime dose could be given as soon as they get home from school.

Excipients

Where possible use sugar-free preparations, particularly for long-term medication. The BNFC states which branded preparations are sugar-free. Some liquid preparations have a high level of alcohol which is unsuitable for children. Information on excipients is also shown in the BNFC.

Prescribing for patients with liver disease

Drug metabolism occurs mainly, but not exclusively, in the liver; prescribing for patients with liver disease can be difficult. There is no direct measure that allows you to quantify liver function in terms of ability to metabolise drugs. Variation in the type of liver disease and the severity of liver disease will both affect how drug metabolism is altered. This makes it difficult to make definitive dosage recommendations.

How would you adjust doses in liver disease?

The most important indicators of a reduced liver function as far as metabolism is concerned are a raised international normalised ratio (INR) and reduced serum albumin. If this is the case, you may need to consider a reduction of the dose of liver-metabolised drugs.

Sometimes medicines may have been studied in patients with liver disease and there are specific recommendations in the BNF or the SmPC (2023).

Drug choice with regards to complications of liver disease

If you have a patient with liver failure under your care, you are likely to encounter some of the complications of liver disease such as encephalopathy, ascites and variceal bleeding.

You may need to adjust drug therapy if these are present as the side-effect profile of some drugs may have an impact on these complications.

The BNF is a useful source and does give some advice on dose changes for some drugs, but if the specific recommendations for dose or medication change are not in the BNF, it is best to contact your local medicines information unit.

Prescribing for patients with renal impairment

Dose adjustment in renal impairment

The degree of dose adjustment required in renal impairment will depend on the proportion of the drug that is eliminated by the kidneys and the dose-related toxicity. Dose reduction can be achieved by either reducing the dose itself or extending the dosing interval.

How can you estimate renal function?

In order to adjust doses of drugs eliminated by the renal route, you need to be able to quantify the degree of renal impairment. The two most common methods in use are the Chronic Kidney Disease Epidemiology Collaboration (CKD-EPI) formula which leads to the estimated glomerular filtration rate (eGFR) and the Cockcroft and Gault equation, which measures creatinine clearance.

The CKD-EPI formula is the recommended method for estimating GFR and calculating drug doses in most patients with renal impairment. This method is adjusted for BSA and uses serum creatinine, age, sex and race as variables. When sending bloods for estimation of the level of renal function or dysfunction, laboratories should use the CKD-EPI formula to routinely report eGFR.

The formula is shown in the BNF (see **Box 8.2**) in the section on 'Prescribing in renal impairment' and is a laboratory-calculated formula.

Box 8.2 CKD-EPI equation

eGFR (mL/min/1.73m^2) = 141 × min(SCr/K, 1)$^\alpha$ × max(SCr/K, 1)$^{-1.209}$ × 0.993^{Age} [× 1.018 if female] [× 1.159 if black]

Where:
SCr = serum creatinine in mg/dL
K = 0.7 for females and 0.9 for males
α = −0.329 for females and −0.411 for males
min (SCr/K, 1) indicates the minimum of SCr/K or 1
max (SCr/K, 1) indicates the maximum of SCr/K or 1.

Cockcroft and Gault equation: creatinine clearance

The relatively constant rate of production of creatinine in individual patients together with almost exclusive glomerular filtration means that creatinine clearance (CrCl) should reflect GFR and therefore kidney function. Historically, the Cockcroft and Gault formula (**Box 8.3**) is the most established formula for estimating creatinine clearance. However, the eGFR is now used widely.

Box 8.3 Cockcroft and Gault formula

$$\text{CrCl (mL/min)} = \frac{(140\text{-age}) \times \text{weight (kg)} \times F}{\text{Serum Creatinine (micromol/L)}}$$

F = 1.04 female, 1.23 male. Use ideal body weight if obese.

The Cockcroft and Gault formula measures creatinine clearance and is not equivalent to eGFR. It is used for estimating renal function and calculating drug doses in elderly patients or patients at extremes of muscle mass.

Prescribing in pregnancy

Drugs can have harmful effects on the embryo and foetus at any stage (including after birth) yet for some patients denying medication may lead to uncontrolled disease which may be more harmful to both the patient and foetus than the risk of continuing therapy. There may be times when you are asked to prescribe for a pregnant woman, assuming this is within your scope of practice. You will therefore need to make a careful assessment of the risks and benefits to both the patient and foetus. You will also need to consider this if prescribing in women of childbearing age if there is a potential for pregnancy.

Teratogenic effects of drugs

A teratogen is any agent that causes an abnormality following foetal exposure during pregnancy. In the early 1960s, a drug you will know of called thalidomide was used to treat morning sickness. Exposure of the foetus during this early stage of development resulted in cases of phocomelia, a congenital malformation in which the hands and feet are attached to abbreviated arms and legs (Genetic Alliance, 2010).

Assessing the teratogenic risks of medicines, particularly new medicines, is difficult. Ethical issues prevent the inclusion of pregnant patients in clinical trials, therefore most data in humans comes from epidemiological studies and case reports or from animal studies, although extrapolation of results to humans cannot be assumed. For this reason, no drug can be considered safe beyond all doubt, but older drugs tend to be used in preference as there will have been more experience with them.

What factors affect teratogenicity?

There are a number of general principles that affect teratogenicity that can be useful to you when considering any potential risk.

Timing of exposure

The embryonic phase (days 18–55) is the highest risk period. Exposure during this period is most likely to result in malformations. During the foetal period (day 56 to birth), organs continue to develop and some remain susceptible to damage, such as the cerebral cortex and kidneys. Functional abnormalities (e.g., deafness) may also occur. The BNFC states that drugs given shortly before term, or during labour, can have adverse effects on labour or on the neonate after delivery.

The BNF and BNFC identify drugs which may have harmful effects in pregnancy and indicate the trimester of risk, and those drugs which are not known to be harmful in pregnancy. The information is based on human data, but information from animal studies has been included for some drugs when its omission might be misleading. Care is always needed when prescribing for pregnant women, but if particular care is needed, this is indicated under the relevant drug in the BNF and BNFC.

Dose

There is a general recommendation that you should prescribe the lowest effective dose in pregnancy as teratogenic effects may be dose-dependent.

Multiple drug therapy

Risk of teratogenicity may be increased if the number of drugs taken concomitantly is increased.

Maternal pharmacokinetic changes

Significant changes in drug distribution may occur because of an increase of up to 50 per cent in blood volume, and a mean increase of 8 litres in body water. Kidney function also changes, with an increase in glomerular filtration rate of 50 per cent, which may affect drugs that are excreted predominantly by the kidneys. You may need to carry out more frequent monitoring for drugs with narrow therapeutic indices such as digoxin, gentamicin, carbamazepine, phenytoin, lithium and theophylline.

Question 8.1

What are the key principles for reducing risk in pregnancy?

Think about what should be considered, avoided and assessed if prescribing for a pregnant woman.

Answer 8.1

Key principles for reducing risk in pregnancy:

- only consider using a medicine when it is really needed;
- assess risk–benefit – the risk of exposure of the foetus must be balanced against the risk of uncontrolled disease if therapy is stopped;
- consider non-drug treatments where possible and only prescribe drugs if essential;
- if possible, avoid all drug use during the first trimester;
- avoid new drugs – there is usually little information available on their safety in pregnancy;
- avoid multiple drug therapy;
- avoid known teratogens in women of childbearing age; if this is not possible, the potential risks should be discussed with the patient;
- use the lowest effective dose for as short a period as possible;
- consider the need for therapeutic drug monitoring and dose alteration for drugs with narrow therapeutic index;
- avoid alcohol, tobacco and other recreational substances.

See, Russel, 2021.

Sources of information

Prescribing in pregnancy is discussed in the section at the beginning of the BNF called 'Guidance on prescribing'. The BNF also gives brief information on use in pregnancy under individual drug monographs. The SmPC (2023) may give more information but may tend to err on the side of caution. You can obtain detailed information from the UK Teratology Information Service, the telephone number and web address of which can be found on the inside cover of the BNF and BNFC or from your local medicines information services.

There are two very important reports mentioned and summarised in the BNF and which should be read prior to prescribing for women who may be considering pregnancy, those who are pregnant or for those who are breast-feeding.

For those considering becoming pregnant and who are on particular medicines, see MHRA, 2019. For those who are pregnant or are considering breast-feeding, see MHRA, 2021.

Prescribing for breast-feeding women

The NHS has produced a document about the benefits of breast-feeding (NHS, 2020), but the section on medicine use is brief. Any mother who is breast-feeding or wants to breast-feed is likely to ask you about any issues with medicines she is taking or about to take. You need to understand where to find information and what action may be necessary. It will still be the mother's decision but you can arm them with as much information as possible. This will ensure that infants are protected from adverse drug reactions from the mother's prescribed medicines and equally that both necessary maternal medication and breast-feeding can continue wherever possible. Most drugs pass into breast milk to some degree, though the overall dose that the infant receives is normally low and usually below a therapeutic level for the infant. The BNF is, as usual an excellent source of first-line information. Under each medicine is a guide to patients who are pregnant or who are breast-feeding, which can help you decide if you need further information.

What factors affect infant risk?

There are a number of factors which affect the risk of an infant being exposed to drugs from breast.

Infant maturity

As discussed in the section on prescribing in children, neonates and premature infants will not have fully developed kidney and liver function needed for elimination and metabolism of drugs, and therefore are more at risk of accumulating drugs ingested via breast milk.

Adverse drug reaction profile

The side-effects of the drug are the main factor when you are assessing risk. Of particular concern are cytotoxic drugs and iodine-containing drugs. Combination therapy with drugs with similar side-effects will also be of concern as these effects may be additive – for example, antipsychotic therapy and antiepileptics.

Question 8.2

What general principles should the pregnant woman follow?

Answer 8.2

General principles you should follow to try and minimise the infant's exposure (remember, most medicines can be used throughout breast-feeding; in some cases further risk-reducing methods may be required):

- avoid unnecessary maternal use – in particular avoid complementary and alternative medication because of a lack of data, and advise mothers to seek advice before purchasing any over the counter (OTC) products;
- multiple medication regimens may pose an increased risk, especially when adverse effects such as drowsiness are additive;
- assess risk–benefit in individual cases – consider particular risk factors such as infant prematurity and multiple maternal medicines. Consult specialist information sources if necessary (see below);
- minimise exposure – use the lowest effective dose for the shortest possible time;
- consider local therapy (e.g., topical/inhaled) which normally results in lower maternal plasma levels and therefore lower passage into milk;
- if the drug has a short half-life, advise taking the dose immediately after feeding to avoid feeding at peak milk concentrations;
- medicines with a long half-life can increase the risk of accumulation in the infant and therefore increase the risk of adverse effects;
- where appropriate, avoid drugs with toxic side-effects in adults or children (e.g., cytotoxics);
- or withhold breast-feeding until after a suitable washout period of the medicine (this is most appropriate for short courses of a hazardous medicine);
- avoid new drugs – older drugs are more likely to have data to guide use in breast-feeding;
- monitor the infant for adverse effects.

(Chapman, 2022)

Sources of information

As mentioned above, the BNF gives brief information on medicines use in breast milk under individual drug monographs. It identifies drugs that should be used with caution or are contraindicated in breast-feeding; that can be given to the mother during breast-feeding because they are present in milk in amounts which are too small to be harmful to the infant; or that might be present in milk in significant amounts but are not known to be harmful.

The SmPC (2023) for each drug will again tend to err on the side of caution. Your local medicines information service will be able to give you more detailed advice where BNF advice is not definitive or too brief.

The reports noted above from the MHRA (2021) are repeated in the section on breast-feeding in the BNF.

Prescribing for older people

Have a look at the section of the BNF entitled 'Prescribing in the elderly' (bnf.nice.org.uk/guidance/prescribing-in-the-elderly.html). This gives a short overview of the issues around prescribing for this group.

In particular, there is a section entitled 'STOPP (Screening Tool of Older Persons, potentially inappropriate Prescriptions) and START (Screening Tool to Alert to Right Treatment) criteria'. These are evidence-based criteria used to review medication regimens in elderly people. The STOPP criteria (Gallagher et al., 2008) aims to reduce the incidence of medicines-related adverse events from potentially inappropriate prescribing and polypharmacy. START (O'Mahony et al., 2015) can be used to prevent omissions of indicated, appropriate medicines in older patients with specific conditions.

Age UK estimates that almost 2 million people over 65 are likely to be taking at least seven prescribed medicines. This number doubles to approaching 4 million for those taking at least five medicines. In England overall more than one in ten people aged over 65 takes at least eight different prescribed medications weekly. This high prevalence of medication use, together with comorbidity and changes in pharmacokinetics and pharmacodynamics increases the risk of encountering adverse drug reactions and drug interactions when you prescribe for this patient group (Age UK, 2019).

What pharmacokinetic changes take place in the older person?

As you know from Chapter 6, pharmacokinetics describes how the body handles medicines. Important age-related changes occur principally with distribution, excretion and metabolism. Drenth-van Maanen et al.'s article (2019) summarises the various pharmacokinetic changes that may affect medicine-taking.

Activity 8.2

Look up digoxin in the BNF – what advice is given under cautions for dosing in older people? What might this advice mean to you in clinical practice?

Distribution

With increasing age, the proportion of body fat increases and the proportion of body water decreases. This means that for water-soluble drugs, the smaller proportion of body water means that the same dose of say, digoxin, results in higher serum levels in older people and, as you saw from Activity 8.2, the dose of digoxin should be reduced in older people.

For fat-soluble drugs with the larger proportion of body fat, the main result is that the half-life increases and it takes longer to clear a dose from the body, with an increased risk of accumulation. An example of this is nitrazepam. This is a long-acting benzodiazepine, and the half-life increases from approximately 30 to 40 hours in the older person, making it an inappropriate choice for night sedation as significant drug levels are still likely to be present the following morning, which may increase the risk of falls and confusion. In practice you may notice that long-acting benzodiazepines such as nitrazepam are still prescribed for older people. All are listed in the STOPP criteria.

Excretion

As you saw from the section on pharmacokinetics, the principal organ responsible for excretion of medicines in the body is the kidney. With increasing age, renal function declines. This affects the clearance of many drugs such as water-soluble antibiotics, diuretics, digoxin, water-soluble beta blockers, lithium, nonsteroidal anti-inflammatory drugs and the direct oral anticoagulants (DOACs), such as dabigatran, rivaroxaban and apixaban.

Comorbidities such as heart failure or diabetes can also worsen renal function, making it important to check and monitor renal function in older people and adjust doses accordingly. See the section on renal impairment for how to do this in practice and Drenth-van Maanen et al. (2019), mentioned above.

Metabolism

Although there is an age-related decline in hepatic blood and liver volume, the large reserve of the liver means that you are unlikely to need to adjust doses of medicines metabolised in the liver unless there is evidence of actual liver disease or severe dysfunction. However, the activity of drug metabolism enzymes in the liver is decreased so that the half-life of the drug may be prolonged.

What pharmacodynamic changes take place in the older person?

In general, older people have increased sensitivity to medicines, even allowing for the changes in serum levels that may occur as a result of pharmacokinetic changes described above. Most commonly this is due to a decline in homeostatic reserve. Some common examples are given below.

Postural hypotension

The normal homeostatic response to maintain blood pressure on standing is tachycardia and vasoconstriction, both of which may be impaired in older people. Medicines that inhibit this response are more likely to produce postural hypotension which may increase the risk of falls. Examples include antihypertensive agents and medicines with vasodilatory side-effects (e.g., calcium channel blockers, nitrates and alpha blockers). Falls in older people are a major cause of morbidity and mortality, and national guidance recommends that you should review medicines that may have contributed to falls as part of a wider multifactorial assessment in those who fall (NICE, 2017).

Cognitive function

Medicines that act on the CNS such as antidepressants and anxiolytics may worsen cognitive function, particularly where there is pre-existing cognitive impairment. Opiates which are taken regularly by elderly people can also have an effect. Cholinergic transmission is considered to play an important role in cognitive function, with the result that medicines with anticholinergic side-effects (e.g., oxybutynin, hyoscine and amitriptyline) may lead to confusion in older people. If you see older people who appear confused, you should always review their medicines as potential side-effects of existing medication.

Other risk factors for medicine-related problems in older people

Recent discharge from hospital

This is a high-risk period as changes to medicines may frequently have been made, both intentional and unintentional. Good communication between secondary and primary care is essential. This should include what medicines have been started and stopped, reasons for these changes and instructions for any ongoing monitoring.

Poor vision and hearing can affect the ability of patients to receive and use information about how to take medicines correctly. Patient information leaflets that come with dispensed medicines are often in a small font size. Larger print leaflets are available from the EMC website. More information about this can be found at www.medicines.org.uk/emc/xpil

Physical dexterity

It is not only older people who experience difficulty in opening blister packs and 'child-proof' medicine bottles, but the issue may be more common in this group of patients. Inhaler use may also be difficult. Therefore, you need to ensure the patient is able to access and use the medicines you are prescribing. You may find it useful to liaise with the pharmacy with regards to assessing patients' ability to access and use their medicines and providing advice and alternatives.

Summary

This chapter considered prescribing within the following patient groups: children, patients with hepatic impairment, patients with renal impairment, pregnant women, breast-feeding women and older people. It looked at each group individually and considered any changes in pharmacokinetics and dynamics. For each group key information sources guiding appropriate drug choice and dose have been highlighted.

References

Age UK 2019. *Age UK Calls for a More Considered Approach to Prescribing Medicines for Older People*. Available at www.ageuk.org.uk/latest-press/articles/2019/august/age-uk-calls-for-a-more-considered-approach-to-prescribing-medicines-for-older-people/ (accessed May 2022).

Batchelor, H.K. and Marriott, F.J. 2015. Paediatric pharmacokinetics. *British Journal of Clinical Pharmacology*. **79**(3), pp. 395–404. Available at www.ncbi.nlm.nih.gov/pmc/

articles/PMC4345950/#:~:text=Elimination%20of%20drugs%20and%20their,the%20 first%20year%20of%20life (accessed May 2022).

BNF 2023. *British National Formulary.* London: BMA and RPS. Available at bnf.nice.org.uk/ (accessed May 2023).

BNFC 2023. *British National Formulary for Children.* London: BMJ, Pharmaceutical Press and RCPCH. Available at bnf.nice.org.uk/ (accessed May 2023).

Chapman, V. 2022. *Advising on Medicines During Breastfeeding.* Specialist Pharmacy Services. Available at www.sps.nhs.uk/articles/advising-on-medicines-during-breastfeeding/ (accessed 30 May 2023).

Department of Health (DoH) 2005. *The National Service Framework for Renal Services Part Two: Chronic Kidney Disease, Acute Renal Failure and End of Life Care.* Available at assets. publishing.service.gov.uk/government/uploads/system/uploads/attachment_data/ file/199002/National_Service_Framework_for_Renal_Services_Part_Two_-_Chronic_ Kidney_Disease__Acute_Renal_Failure_and_End_of_Life_Care.pdf (accessed May 2022).

Drenth-van Maanen, A.C., Wilting, I. and Jansen, P.A.F. 2019. Prescribing medicines to older people: How to consider the impact of ageing on human organ and body functions. *British Journal of Clinical Pharmacology.* **86**(10), pp. 1921–30. Available at doi.org/10.1111/bcp.14094 (accessed 30 May 2023).

Gallagher, P., Ryan, C., Byrne, S., Kennedy, J. and O'Mahony, D. 2008. STOPP and START: Consensus validation. *International Journal of Clinical Pharmacology and Therapeutics.* **46**(2), pp. 72–83.

Genetic Alliance 2010. *Understanding Genetics: A District of Columbia Guide for Patients and Health Professionals.* Washington, DC: District of Columbia Department of Health. Available at pubmed.ncbi.nlm.nih.gov/23586106/ (accessed May 2022).

MHRA/CHM 2019. *Medicines with Teratogenic Potential: What is Effective Contraception and How Often is Pregnancy Testing Needed?* Available at www.gov.uk/drug-safety-update/ medicines-with-teratogenic-potential-what-is-effective-contraception-and-how-often-is-pregnancy-testing-needed (accessed May 2022).

MHRA/CHM 2021. *Medicines in Pregnancy and Breastfeeding: New Initiative for Consistent Guidance: Report on Optimising Data for Medicines Used During Pregnancy.* Available at www.gov.uk/drug-safety-update/medicines-in-pregnancy-and-breastfeeding-new-initiative-for-consistent-guidance-report-on-optimising-data-for-medicines-used-during-pregnancy (accessed May 2022).

NHS 2020. *Benefits of Breastfeeding.* Available at www.nhs.uk/conditions/baby/breastfeeding-and-bottle-feeding/breastfeeding/benefits/ (accessed August 2022).

NICE 2017. Falls in older people. Quality standard [QS86]. *Falls in Older People: Assessing Risk and Prevention.* Clinical guideline [CG161]. Available at www.nice.org.uk/guidance/ cg161 (accessed 20 September 2023).

O'Mahony, D., O'Sullivan, D., Byrne, S., O'Connor, M.N., Ryan, C. and Gallagher, P. 2015. STOPP/START criteria for potentially inappropriate prescribing in older people version 2. *Age and Ageing.* **44**(2), pp. 213–18.

RPS 2021. *A Competency Framework for All Prescribers.* Available at www.rpharms.com/resources/ frameworks/prescribing-competency-framework/competency-framework (accessed 12 May 2023).

Russel, P. 2021. *The Principles of Prescribing in Pregnancy.* Specialist Pharmacy Services. Available at www.sps.nhs.uk/articles/the-principles-of-prescribing-in-pregnancy/ (accessed 30 May 2023).

SmPC 2023. *Electronic Medicines Compendium.* Available at www.medicines.org.uk (accessed 30 May 2023).

9

Adverse Drug Reactions and Interactions

Barry Strickland-Hodge

Chapter summary

- This chapter will consider two important aspects of prescribing: adverse drug reactions (ADEs, ADRs and SEs) and drug interactions.

Introduction

The *Competency Framework for All Prescribers* (RPS, 2021) Competency 4, Prescribe, has the supporting statements 4.1: 'Prescribes a medicine or device with up-to-date awareness of its actions, indications, dose, contraindications, interactions, cautions and adverse effects' and 4.2: 'Understands the potential for adverse effects and takes steps to recognise, and manage them, whilst minimising risk'.

In Competency 6, Monitor and review, supporting statement 6.4 states: 'Recognises and reports suspected adverse events to medicines and medical devices using appropriate reporting systems'.

Adverse Drug Events (ADE), Adverse Drug Reactions (ADR) and Side-Effects (SE)

The previous two chapters looked at medicines which require particular care when prescribing, based on reports to the MHRA, and also prescribing for specific patient groups. Whatever care is taken, major or minor side-effects are possible with any medicine.

The terminology used can be confusing and is often used inappropriately. The three main terms used are adverse drug events (ADE), adverse drug reactions (ADR) and side-effects (SE). They can be defined in various ways but the most usual are shown in **Box 9.1**.

Box 9.1 What is the difference between an ADE, ADR and SE?

ADE

An adverse drug event is 'an injury resulting from the use of a drug. Under this definition, the term ADE includes harm caused by the drug (adverse drug reactions and overdoses) and harm from the use of the drug (including dose reductions and discontinuations of drug therapy)' (Nebeker et al., 2004). An easy-to-read set of definitions can be found at: www.pbm.va.gov/PBM/vacenterformedicationsafety/tools/AdverseDrugReaction.pdf Adverse drug event is the overarching term.

ADR

An adverse drug reaction is a 'response to a drug which is noxious and unintended, and which occurs at doses normally used in man for prophylaxis, diagnosis, or therapy of disease or for the modification of physiologic function' (WHO, 1969). ADRs are not the same as overdoses because, looking at the definition again, ADRs occur at normal doses. An overdose could be covered by the term ADE.

Side-Effect (SE)

A side-effect is an undesired effect that occurs when the medication is administered, regardless of the dose. Unlike adverse events, side-effects are mostly foreseen by the prescriber and the patient is told to be aware of the effects that could happen while on the therapy. The term 'side-effect' tends to normalise the concept of injury from drugs. It has been recommended that this term should generally be avoided in favour of ADR. However, the BNF uses the term 'side-effects' currently. Some side-effects might be useful. For example, a side-effect of an antihistamine such as chlorphenamine is drowsiness; so, if you have a rash that itches and you take it at night, it may help reduce the itch and the drowsiness may help you to sleep.

ADRs are different from side-effects and are never desired; they require interventions such as changing or stopping the medication, whereas most side-effects spontaneously resolve with time. The two words are often incorrectly used interchangeably.

ADRs can have a major impact on patients – not only on their recovery time and general wellbeing, but also in the confidence they have in your ability to prescribe safely. Some ADRs can be predicted by their pharmacology but others are more subtle and affect only some people.

Other potential issues with ADRs are that they can cause hospital admission, complicate existing diseases or delay their cure; they can mimic other diseases leading to possible additional unnecessary treatment; they can affect a patient's quality of life; and all potentially cost a great deal of money.

What is the frequency of ADRs that lead to hospital admission?

Research into the frequency of ADRs that lead to hospital admission varies depending on the study design and how ADR is defined. Some studies and systematic reviews suggest that the rate of hospital admissions directly due to ADRs is 5 per cent, which I am sure you will agree is high. A very well-respected, large prospective observational study in Merseyside found 6.5 per cent of admissions were due to ADRs (Pirmohamed et al., 2004). It is much more difficult to estimate the level of ADRs in the community as reporting is not as efficient and trials are more difficult to conduct, but they are important and do cause problems to patients.

Activity 9.1

Before reading further into this chapter, find the sections in the BNF or in the electronic BNF (www.bnf.org) that discusses ADRs. There is a general section near the beginning of the BNF and there are also sections on ADRs in the children and elderly prescribing sections. It is possible to have an adverse reaction to a medical device such as intrauterine devices and there is a short section to guide you as to how to report these.

Classification of ADRs according to incidence

The frequency and type of side-effects differs, of course, but the commonly used guide is the European classification of ADRs.

European legislation brought in a simple classification according to incidence of reported ADRs. This terminology is used in the SmPC, which was mentioned in Chapter 2 of this book. You can find the SmPCs at www.medicines.org.uk. The classification is shown in **Box 9.2**.

Box 9.2   European classification of ADRs according to incidence

Very common	More than 10%	(>1 in 10)
Common	1–10%	(1 in 100 to 1 in 10)
Uncommon	0.1–1%	(1 in 1,000 to 1 in 100)
Rare	0.01–0.1%	(1 in 10,000 to 1 in 1,000)
Very rare	Less than 0.01%	(<1 in 10,000)

Classification of ADRs by definition

ADRs are divided into two main groups: Type A and Type B (Rawlins and Thompson, 1977).

Type A

Type A ADRs are relatively common and are often discovered during the clinical trials phase of drug development. They are usually related to the pharmacological properties of the drug and occur at normal doses in average people. They can manifest as additive effects to the original drug effect, thus the name Type A or 'Augmented' ADRs. They can often be predicted, so warning of their possibility can be given to patients with guidance as to what to do if they occur. These warnings are on the patient information leaflet that accompanies the dispensed medicine. Illness or symptoms can be high, with gastrointestinal disorders common side-effects, but mortality is low. Examples of Type A ADRs might be constipation with opioids due to their action on the gut; dry mouth and blurred vision with tricyclic antidepressants because of their antimuscarinic effects.

Type B

Type B ADRs, are not predictable, which leads to their definition as Type B or 'Bizarre'. When the reason for the ADR is found to be genetic, the ADR is often called a pharmaco-genetic reaction. Type B ADRs include allergic reactions or genetic responses – for example, rashes with penicillins. Awareness of such rashes is quite high, and also that anaphylaxis is a potential issue.

Over the years additional 'refinements' to the initial classification have been made. For example, you can now read about **Types C** (chronic, develops after chronic use); **D** (delayed, occurs long after use); **E** (end of use, effects after stopping the medicine); and **F** (failure of therapy, where the medication does not resolve the condition for which it was prescribed). You might consider this last one, F, as not an ADR at all, but it is referred to (Edwards and Aronson, 2000). However, A and B are the most important.

Serious ADRs

Serious ADRs are defined, not surprisingly, as those that prove fatal; are life-threatening; are disabling or incapacitating; result in or prolong hospitalisation; produce congenital abnormalities or are considered medically significant (MHRA, Yellow Card; see yellowcard.mhra.gov.uk/definitions/ for further information).

As a prescriber, you must report *ALL* potential ADRs for new drugs which are being monitored by the MHRA. These are indicated by an inverted black triangle ▼next to the drug's name in the BNF. In BNF 82, in the Contraception section, there is a black triangle against the intra-uterine device Jaydess, which contains 13.5mg levonorgestrel, manufactured by Bayer. In the EMC, under the same brand name, you see it says, '▼This medicine is subject to additional monitoring. This will allow quick identification of new safety information. Healthcare professionals are asked to report any suspected adverse reactions' (EMC, Jaydess, updated July 2022). Note that these will change depending on the edition of the BNF and any updates of the EMC as they remain only while the MHRA is monitoring the particular drug or device.

ADRs as potential symptoms of other conditions

Above, we said that ADRs could mimic other conditions leading to possible additional unnecessary treatment. So, at the consultation, the potential that a symptom, described by the patient, could be an ADR to something the patient is currently taking needs to be considered by taking a careful medication history, including OTC and even borrowed or bought-online medicines. You should consider ADRs as part of the differential diagnosis of any newly presented condition.

How can you reduce the risk of ADRs?

Knowing the type of patients or conditions that might predispose a patient to suffer an ADR and knowing the type of drugs that cause most ADRs will help you when you are prescribing. Make sure the dose and drug choice are appropriate for the age, condition and weight of the patient. Always discuss the possibility of side-effects with patients and listen and react to their concerns. If the patient decides to continue treatment, ensure they receive counselling on correct use of medicines and what to do if they do suspect side-effects.

Remember, always take or refer to a detailed drug history when starting a new drug, including any previous ADRs; stop drugs that are no longer necessary. This is important when you consider those medicines that are on the patient's repeat prescribing list. Some patients may request all of the medicines each month or two, though they may only use some of them. Ask, in a non-judgemental way, about this. You can then decide if the new symptom is an ADR and also if the new medicine is likely to interact with any of the patient's repeat list. Before you prescribe, ensure the patient understands the likely benefits of the medication but also the risks associated. You could use the patient information leaflet (PIL) to inform your discussions. These can be accessed on www.medicines.org.uk

Patients may not be aware that the generic drug they are being given by you is the same as the brand drug they got some years ago and reacted badly to. People forget! It should be in the notes.

Patients who may be more susceptible to ADRs

Chapter 8 has already discussed prescribing for special patient groups (and see Ferner, 2019). For susceptibility, consider the age of the patient, where the very old and the very young are at greater risk; gender where it appears that women are more susceptible to ADRs (Drici and Clément, 2001), patients with renal, hepatic or cardiac disease; patients with known abnormal metabolism; genetic differences such as patients with glucose-6-phosphate dehydrogenase deficiency (G6PD) and polypharmacy – these are some of the areas to consider before prescribing (Lee, 2006).

Which drugs potentially cause more ADRs?

There are over a billion prescription items issued in England alone each year. With such a large number of prescription medicines being issued to patients the potential for ADRs is high. Most prescriptions are issued in the community and NSAIDs are the most common drug group for the reporting of ADRs. Other drugs and drug groups were discussed in more detail in Chapter 7, which covers which medicines have the potential for serious problems and are likely to produce more ADRs.

How do you report ADRs?

Thalidomide was developed in the 1950s as a sedative or tranquiliser. It was found useful in other conditions too, including morning sickness in pregnant women. As you know, the drug caused foetal abnormalities and serious birth defects. Following the realisation that it was thalidomide taken by the pregnant woman that was causing this ADR, a surveillance system was set up in 1964 which is still the main method of collating ADRs in the UK. It is usually called the Yellow Card system of reporting. Anyone can send in a Yellow Card or complete one online – not only healthcare professionals, but also patients and the pharmaceutical industry.

The Yellow Card scheme has had a major impact on the labelling, warnings and availability of drugs following investigation of reports of suspected ADRs. Drugs can be withdrawn, although this is more often as a result of the pharmaceutical company removing the drug from the market voluntarily.

You can find out more about how drug surveillance and Yellow Card reports are used to develop knowledge about safe use of drugs by signing up on the MHRA website to receive their monthly *Drug Safety Update*. To report a suspected ADR, take a look at the new Yellow Card reporting site: yellowcard.mhra.gov.uk/

Looking at ADR reports

To see if a drug you use has had ADRs reported you can use the MHRA website, www.medicines.org.uk, for suspected ADRs. The MHRA publishes this information in the form of interactive drug analysis profiles (iDAPs). There is an iDAP for each licensed medicines by drug substance. Within an iDAP you can see all suspected ADRs which are reported to the MHRA. For example, look up ramipril on www.gov.uk/drug-analysis-prints. Go to the page which shows the iDAP for ramipril: there is a full breakdown of the ADRs reported to the MHRA. You will see the following.

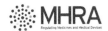
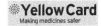

Interactive Drug Analysis Profile

Overview

This Interactive Drug Analysis profile (DAP) displays an overview of all UK spontaneous suspected Adverse Drug Reactions (ADRs) reported through the Yellow Card Scheme. It is important to note that reported adverse reactions have not been proven to be related to the drug, and should not be interpreted as a list of known side effects. The MHRA encourages the use of Yellow Card data, however to ensure that it is interpreted in the correct way please refer to the guidance at the bottom of this page. Definitions and an explanation of terms used can also be found in the glossary page.

RAMIPRIL
- Single constituent brand names: ACCORD HEALTHCARE RAMIPRIL, ACCORD-UK RAMIPRIL, ALTACE, APS TEVA RAMIPRIL, BRISTOL LABS RAMIPRIL, BROWN & BURK RAMIPRIL, CRESCENT PHARMA RAMIPRIL, ENNOGEN PHARMA RAMIPRIL, GENERICS UK RAMIPRIL, MILPHARM RAMIPRIL, RAMIC, RAMIPRIL [not otherwise coded], TEVA UK RAMIPRIL, TRITACE, WOCKHARDT UK RAMIPRIL, ZENTIVA PHARMA UK RAMIPRIL
- Multiple constituent brand names: AVENTIS PHARMA TRITACE, SANDOZ LTD RAMIPRIL, TRIAPIN

- Total number of reactions: 13679 - Total number of ADR reports: 6249
- Total number of serious ADR reports: 4041 - Total number of fatal ADR reports: 66
- Displays show a breakdown of all 6249 UK spontaneous reports received for RAMIPRIL.
- Reports processed up to: 31-Jan-2023

Figure 9.1 Interactive drug analysis profile (iDAP)

Note: Reproduced with kind permission of the MHRA under the terms of the Open Government Licence (OGL) v3.0.

The first report was in 1990, over 30 years ago; there have been 3,848 serious reports since then. However, the MHRA points out on each iDAP that conclusions on the safety and risks of medicines cannot be made on the data shown in the iDAP alone. For comprehensive information about the risks of particular medicines, you should refer to the SmPC at www.medicines.org.uk

The process for reporting an ADR

The process should be simple if it is to encourage more reports. The simplest method is to use the online reporting system at yellowcard.mhra.gov.uk/; you need to register with the MHRA once only.

You do not have to prove causality of any ADR; a suspicion is all that is necessary, particularly for a new drug. If the drug has an inverted triangle next to it in the BNF (see above) you should report any suspected ADR. It does not matter how inconsequential you think the effect actually is as this helps build up a post-marketing picture of the new drug.

Second, report any *serious* potential ADR (see the definition above) whether the drug is new or established. The reason the MHRA continue to request reports for established drugs is they may highlight previously unrecognised effects. For example, Reye's syndrome (a very rare disorder that can cause serious liver and brain damage) was associated with aspirin in teenage children eight decades after it was first marketed. Reye's syndrome mainly affects children and young adults under 20 years of age (NHS Health A–Z, 2019).

Sending the report may allow advice to be given on risk factors for patients such as age or concurrent disease; or how medicines can be used more safely. It cannot be stressed enough how important completing the Yellow Card scheme forms can be.

Drug interactions

You have now read about pharmacology divided into pharmacokinetics (kinetics) and pharmacodynamics (dynamics) (see Chapter 6). The first part of this chapter looked at ADRs; this part looks at drug interactions. You will see that a basic knowledge of dynamics and kinetics will help you understand the mechanism of drug interactions.

Medicines taken by your patients can interact with other prescribed or bought medicines, food, herbs and even biochemical tests.

The effects of one drug on another can be to augment its effect, in other words be additive, potentially leading to toxic levels, or it might prevent its absorption and reduce its activity. In this chapter we will look at the different types of drug interaction to help you become more aware of how to reduce their impact or eliminate them altogether.

What is a drug interaction?

> **Box 9.3**
>
> The current BNF (bnf.nice.org.uk/interactions/appendix-1-interactions/) states:
>
> Two or more drugs given at the same time can exert their effects independently or they can interact. Many interactions are harmless, and even those that are potentially harmful can often be managed, allowing the drugs to be used safely together. Potentially harmful drug interactions may occur in only a small number of patients, but the true incidence is often hard to establish. Furthermore, the severity of a harmful interaction is likely to vary from one patient to another. [As with ADRs, see the previous section] patients at increased risk from drug interactions include the elderly and those with impaired renal or hepatic function.

It is important to be able to use the BNF as a guide to drug interactions and to recognise the main types and mechanisms of such interactions. As with ADRs, certain groups of patients may be more susceptible than others and therefore need to be treated with even more care when prescribing a new drug. Patients taking many medicines will potentially have greater chance of interactions.

If the watchwords for ADRs are: 'always consider an adverse drug reaction as part of your differential diagnosis', then, similarly, with drug interactions, 'always consider side-effects or new symptoms as possibly the result of a drug interaction'.

What is the incidence of drug interactions?

Drug interactions can occur with a prescribed drug and something the patient may have bought OTC or borrowed from a neighbour. They may also occur between a prescribed drug and a herbal medicine the patient has bought, or a food or drink such as grapefruit or cranberry juice. These are difficult to pick up in any study. The estimates for the incidence of drug interactions relate, in many ways, to the number of medicines a patient is taking – polypharmacy.

Some interactions may be good if it means you can take a lower dose of one medicine by taking a second one. It has been suggested that some patients will suffer an interaction with two drugs when another patient will not (Stockley, 2019). Overall, it is a much less clear picture than with ADRs.

Where do you go for information about drug interactions?

Using the BNF as a guide

Whether you use the electronic version of the BNF, an app on your phone or the hard copy, the first place to look for drug interactions is Appendix 1 of the BNF.

Activity 9.2

Look at a current edition of the hard copy version of the BNF and find Appendix 1. This is simply to show you where it is in the BNF and how it is arranged. The app or online will get you there much more quickly. As an example, look at ramipril as we have done previously.

Answer 9.2

Once you have found ramipril, you will see it says 'see ACE inhibitors' as ramipril is a member of this wider group. When you find ACE inhibitors it suggests you look at the tables which appear before the Interactions appendix. Under that there is a list of medicines that can interact with ACE inhibitors. There are various words to indicate the severity of the interaction – avoid, moderate, severe and theoretical – and then another word to indicate the type of evidence to support it. Some, you will see, are based on studies but are anecdotal; however, if they occur they can be severe. For example, under ACE inhibitors there is an entry that says: 'ACE inhibitors are predicted to increase the concentration of lithium. Monitor and adjust dose; Severe but anecdotal'. If you then look up lithium as its own entry there is the entry again under ACE inhibitors. Quite a difficult search for what might be very important.

Using the online version of the BNF (bnf.nice.org.uk/):

From the introductory page there is a box saying Interactions, check for drug interactions. It includes information on the severity of an interaction and the type of evidence to support it. Then it goes on to say: 'View interactions A to Z'. Click that and choose R for ramipril. It shows all of the potential drug interactions in alphabetical order so lithium is easily found with the same advice – but a much simpler way of finding it.

The SmPC (www.medicines.org.uk) has a section (always numbered 4.5) called Interaction with other medicinal products and other forms of interaction. Looking for the same potential drug interaction with lithium, the SmPC states:

'Lithium salts: Excretion of lithium may be reduced by ACE inhibitors and therefore lithium toxicity may be increased. Lithium level must be monitored'.

It does not mention if this is anecdotal.

What are the main types of drug interaction?

The main types of drug interaction are pharmacokinetic in that one drug can affect absorption, distribution, metabolism or excretion of another. In the less common pharmacodynamic interactions, a second drug can affect the way the first drug acts, for example, on receptors.

The most common, clinically significant pharmacokinetic drug interactions relate to metabolism. You were introduced to (or reminded of) pharmacology including pharmacodynamics and pharmacokinetics in Chapter 6.

Pharmacokinetic drug interactions

Remember, pharmacokinetics is the way the body acts on the drug and is made up of absorption, distribution, metabolism and elimination (ADME). In this section we will see how one drug or food could alter one or more of these processes.

Absorption

When you are about to give a new medicine to a patient you need to remember that the new medicine may interact by preventing or even increasing the absorption of one or more of the medicines. The amount and the speed of absorption can be altered by food or other drugs. Gastric emptying could be increased, meaning the medicine could reach the main site of absorption, the small intestine, quicker or it may slow the rate of absorption and more may be destroyed in the stomach. A positive drug interaction could be with metoclopramide, which increases gut motility. If the patient is taking metoclopramide and has a headache and takes paracetamol the action of the metoclopramide on the gut will mean the paracetamol will reach the small intestine more quickly and can have its analgesic effect sooner. Milk and other products containing heavy metals such as calcium, magnesium or aluminium in antacids or food can form what are called chelates, which are insoluble and cannot be absorbed, so some medicines need to be taken on an empty stomach which is usually defined as one hour before or two hours after food.

Distribution

The next pharmacokinetic process in ADME is distribution, although you may argue metabolism should come before distribution. Following absorption, the drug passes to the liver via the hepatic portal vein. There it can be metabolised during first pass. The unmetabolised drug, plus any metabolites, enters the bloodstream and is distributed usually at least partially bound to proteins in the plasma at specific binding sites. If you give a second drug which competes for the same binding sites on the protein, some of the original medicine could be displaced into the plasma. You may remember that only free unbound drug can have an action, so this displacement will increase the amount of free drug. In the past this was thought to be of major significance. However, as the drug is displaced into the plasma it is quickly metabolised. Displacement rarely produces more than transient potentiation because this increased concentration of free drug will usually be eliminated. It is difficult to identify any clinically significant drug interactions specifically due to plasma protein displacement. There is a *potential* issue for drugs that are more than 90 per cent protein-bound, such as warfarin, but this is theoretical. It may be important in therapeutic drug monitoring – for example, with phenytoin and in some cases where the drug is given intravenously.

Metabolism

The liver is the main but not only site of metabolism. From Chapter 6 you will be aware of the importance in metabolism in the liver of the cytochrome P450 enzyme isomers. Some drugs will only be affected by specific cytochrome P450 isoenzymes and not others. One drug may induce the isomer that metabolises another drug (enzyme inducers) the patient is taking which will have the effect of decreasing the amount of the first drug and potentially reduce its clinical effect. Conversely, a drug may inhibit the P450 isomer (enzyme inhibitors) that metabolises another drug the patient is taking resulting in an increase and potential toxic level.

For example, rifampicin is an enzyme inducer. The effectiveness of any drug taken at the same time which is metabolised by the same P450 isomer – such as ciclosporin, an anti-rejection drug – will be reduced and therefore the potential for organ rejection is increased. Rifampicin can also induce the isoenzyme that metabolises oral contraceptives so their effectiveness is potentially reduced which can lead to a failure of the contraceptive; additional contraceptive advice will be required. Drugs that inhibit the cytochrome P450 isoenzymes such as clarithromycin will have the effect of reducing the metabolism of another similarly metabolised drug, leading to an increase in the plasma concentration and potential toxicity.

Elimination

Many drugs and their metabolites, once they have been made soluble by enzyme action, are excreted by the kidneys. If drugs are to be reabsorbed in the kidney tubules, they need to be in a lipid soluble form and unionised. The acidity or alkalinity of urine has a significant influence on drug excretion and reabsorption. Most drugs are either weak acids (such as ibuprofen) or weak bases (such as diazepam). In alkaline urine, acidic drugs are more readily ionised. In acidic urine, alkaline drugs are more readily ionised. Ionised substances are more soluble in water so dissolve in the body fluids more readily for excretion but cannot be reabsorbed so are lost. Therefore, if the pH of the urine is changed by another drug or food this will affect the elimination of that drug.

Drug–food and drug–herb interactions

As mentioned in the section above, the absorption of drugs can be affected by the presence of food, such as milk, where an insoluble chelate can be formed. Other drugs that form chelates with milk and antacids are bisphosphonates and ciprofloxacin. Conversely, some foods can enhance absorption. For example, if the drug requires an acid environment to be absorbed, such as itraconazole, it would be best to take with food.

Activity 9.3

Look at the Interactions section of the BNF in hard copy, online or via the app. What does it say about cranberry juice?

Answer 9.3

The BNF states that cranberry juice increases the anticoagulant effect of coumarins (warfarin), advising that it should be avoided as this can be severe, but adds that this is anecdotal.

Although anecdotal, as the BNF is currently advising you to avoid, it is best to remain cautious.

Now look at grapefruit juice and you will see that there are many more entries with different levels of caution or recommendations. Is this surprising to you? For example, the BNF states that grapefruit juice increases the exposure to simvastatin, advising 'avoid' and 'severe', and adds that this information comes from a study.

As a prescriber you will need to be aware of this so you can advise patients accordingly. Pharmacists will add the warnings and advice to labels when the medicine is dispensed, but verbal emphasis can enhance adherence.

Herbs such as Hypericum perforatum (St John's wort), an enzyme inducer, have been known for some time to interact with oestrogens and progestogens. In the BNF hard copy, the Saint is abbreviated to St in the alphabetical listing, so you find the potential interactions under St John's wort. Note that there are a large number of interacting drugs. Look at the evidence for the potential interactions of St John's wort. This preparation can be bought over the counter and therefore the initial consultation needs to ensure you know what other medicines the patient may be taking and which they may have bought or borrowed. Even though the evidence may be slight, the advice is either to stop the St John's wort or to use another form of contraception (emergency or not) if it is to be continued.

Pharmacodynamic interactions

Remember, pharmacodynamics is the way the drug acts on the body. These are less frequent than pharmacokinetic interactions and may involve competition for receptor sites.

Beta blockers are sometimes used for hypertension; the older ones such as propranolol are not as specific to the Beta 1 receptors in the heart and may have an effect on the Beta 2 receptors. Beta 2 receptors are predominantly present in airway smooth muscle. If the patient is currently using a Beta 2 receptor agonist, such as salbutamol, the propranolol may block the effect so should not be given to patients with, for example, asthma.

Drugs in the same class as another will be potentially additive. For example, alcohol is a central nervous system (CNS) depressant. Alcohol plus any other CNS depressant drug can exhibit additive effects. Although not strictly speaking a drug interaction, it is important to consider when counselling patients on their medicines.

It would be useful for you to refer again to Chapters 7 and 8 on medicines requiring particular care and specialist patient groups, respectively.

Medicines that can affect laboratory test results

There are a number of drugs that can give false positive or false negative test results depending on the amount taken and when. Some, such as cephalosporins, can alter urine glucose and ketone test results. However, detailed information about this is beyond the scope of this book and, in fact, published, readily available data on this type of interaction is difficult to find.

How can you avoid drug interactions?

It is often difficult to predict if a drug interaction could occur, particularly if the patient is buying medicines over the counter or possibly borrowing them from friends or relatives. The discussion at the consultation is very important. However, try to keep the number of medicines a patient takes to a minimum. Second, remember that drugs can interact not only with other drugs, but also food and herbal remedies which patients may be buying for themselves. As much as possible, keep in mind the pharmacology of the medicines you wish to prescribe. Take particular care in the elderly and other specific patient groups and don't forget to review a patient's medicines regularly, removing any that are no longer required (deprescribing) from the repeat list.

Summary

In this chapter we discussed definitions and classifications of adverse drug reactions, including their prevalence and potential outcomes. ADRs are important and lead to a number of potential adverse outcomes. On one hand, it may be that the patient's view of you as the prescriber is diminished and, on the other, they may suffer harm including death. Vigilance is essential to try to avoid ADRs and it is important to remember that any reported symptoms might be the results of an ADR to a prescribed medicine; this should be part of the differential diagnosis.

Finally, we discussed how to report ADRs to improve market surveillance, particularly of new products.

Your goal is to ensure ADRs are kept to a minimum by knowing which type of drugs and which patient groups you should be particularly cautious about; if ADRs happen, you should know how to report them. Drug interactions are important to the prescriber and the patient. The detailed history-taking at the consultation should identify all medicines being taken by the patient, some of which might not have been on the record, such as those bought or borrowed. This part of the chapter looked at types of drug interactions and how they might occur and how they might be prevented. Polypharmacy and age are known to increase the chance of an interaction. Remember, it isn't only medicines that can interact with other medicines; foods and compounds containing aluminium, magnesium and other heavy metals can too. You saw that fruit juices such as cranberry and grapefruit may also be important in drug interactions. You cannot know them all, so know how to use the BNF, in whichever form you choose.

References

Barry, C., Bradley, C.P., Britten, N., Stevenson, F.A. and Barber, N. 2000. Patients' unvoiced agendas in general practice consultations: Qualitative study. *British Medical Journal.* **320**(7244), pp. 1246–50.

BNF 2023. *British National Formulary.* London: BMA and RPS. Available at bnf.nice.org.uk/ (accessed May 2023).

Davies, D.M., Ferner, R.E. and Glanville, H. 1998. *Davies's Textbook of Adverse Drug Reactions.* 5th ed. London: Chapman and Hall Medical.

Drici, M.D. and Clément, N. 2001. Is gender a risk factor for adverse drug reactions? *Drug Safety.* **24**(8), pp. 575–85.

Edwards, I.R. and Aronson, J.K. 2000. Adverse drug reactions: Definitions, diagnosis and management. *Lancet.* **356**, pp. 1255–9.

Ferner, R. 2019. Susceptibility to adverse drug reactions. *British Journal of Clinical Pharmacology.* **85**(10), pp. 2205–12.

Lee, A. 2006. *Adverse Drug Reactions.* 2nd ed. London: Pharmaceutical Press.

Leheny, S. 2017. *Adverse Event: Not the Same as 'Side Effect'.* Available at www.pharmacytimes.com/view/adverse-event-not-the-same-as-side-effect (accessed 30 May 2023).

MHRA 2023. *Drug Safety Update.* Available at www.gov.uk/drug-safety-update (accessed May 2023).

NHS Health A–Z 2019. Reyes syndrome. Available at www.nhs.uk/conditions/reyes-syndrome/ (accessed 30 May 2023).

Nebeker, J.R., Barach, P. and Samore, M.H. 2004. Clarifying adverse drug events: A clinician's guide to terminology, documentation, and reporting. *Annals of Internal Medicine.* **140**, pp. 795–801.

Pirmohamed, M., James, S., Meakin, S., Green, C., Scott, A.K., Walley, T.J., Farrar, K., Park, B.K. and Breckenridge, A.M. 2004. Adverse drug reactions as a cause of admission to hospital: Prospective analysis of 18,820 patients. *BMJ.* **329**, pp. 15–19.

Rawlins, M.D. and Thompson, J.W. 1977. Pathogenesis of adverse drug reactions. In Davies, D.M. (ed.), *Textbook of Adverse Drug Reactions.* 1st ed. Oxford: Oxford University Press, p. 44.

SmPC 2020. *Ramipril 5mg interactions.* Available at www.medicines.org.uk/emc/ product/10153/smpc section 4.5 (accessed March 2023).

Stockley, I. 2019. *Stockley's Drug Interactions.* 12th ed. Preston, C.L. (ed.). London: Pharmaceutical Press.

World Health Organization (WHO) 1969. WHO 1969 WHO technical report series, international drug monitoring – the role of the hospital report of a WHO meeting Geneva https://iris.who.int/bitstream/handle/10665/40747/WHO_TRS_425.pdf?sequenc

10

Prescription Writing, Including Risk of Remote Prescribing

Barry Strickland-Hodge, Melanie McGinlay
and Rebecca Dickinson

Chapter summary

The chapter covers the process of:

- prescription writing;
- prescribing of licensed, unlicensed or off-label medicines;
- prescribing controlled drugs;
- considering when generic prescribing is appropriate and when it is not, branded generics;
- risks associated with prescribing using remote methods such as via the telephone.

Prescription writing

In 1991 the UK government produced an executive letter which was sent to all general practitioners. In this, the then Secretary of State for Health alerted prescribers that the legal responsibility for prescribing lies with the individual who signs the prescription. It remains today that the person who signs the prescription takes the legal responsibility and liability. This is important, particularly when you may receive a letter from a hospital recommending a particular medication for your patient which you agree with. If you sign the prescription it is your responsibility. Think about repeat prescriptions and who signs them. This point was reiterated by NHS England (2018): 'Legal responsibility for prescribing lies with the doctor or health professional who signs the prescription and it is the responsibility of the individual prescriber to prescribe within their own level of competence.'

Within the *Competency Framework* (RPS, 2021), Competency 4, Prescribe, has the supporting statement 4.9: 'Electronically generates and/or writes legible, unambiguous and complete prescriptions which meet legal requirements'. The nature of those legal requirements will be discussed in this section.

In the *British National Formulary* (BNF, 2022), near the beginning of the hard copy or online, there is a section called 'Prescription writing' which gives the specific requirements for you, as the prescriber, to create a legal prescription. One of the things that is new since nurses, pharmacists and other healthcare professionals have become prescribers is that it is important to show the type of prescriber who is signing the prescription. The prescription must be signed in ink; electronic facsimile signatures are not acceptable. However, within the Electronic Prescription Service (EPS), prescriptions must be generated and signed electronically by a prescriber before being sent to a patient's nominated pharmacy. The age and the date of birth of the patient should preferably be stated, but it's a legal requirement if the prescription is for a prescription-only medicine for a child under 12 years of age. Prescriptions for controlled drugs (CDs) have some specific legal requirements which will be discussed later. There are occasions when it is important to state the weight of the child so that the dose can be carefully calculated; however, this is not common in primary care. You will need to state the strength of the tablet, capsules, lozenge or liquid and also the quantity required. Try not to use decimal points when they are unnecessary; the BNF gives an example to write 3mg not 3.0mg as it could be mistaken for 30mg. It also advises that quantities less than a gram should be written as mg – for example, if it was 500 milligrams this should be written as 500mg not 0.5g. If you are writing a prescription where the doses are in micrograms the word microgram needs to be written out in full so anything less than 1 milligram needs to be written as micrograms. If you wish to write half a millilitre (mL) this needs to be written as 0.5mL with a zero at the beginning to distinguish it from 5mL if the 0 was missing. If you are intending to write 'as required' as the dose it is recommended that you put a minimum dose interval. You could write 'as required up to four times a day', for example, or 'no more than so many tablets or capsules in 24 hours'.

If your patient is a child it is important to specify the dose in terms of the strength and the dose interval, so if it was for something like amoxicillin oral suspension 125 milligrams in 5 mL you should state 125 milligrams, for example, three times a day not 5mL three times a day. If a dose of an oral medicine is less than 5mL, an oral syringe will be supplied by the pharmacy unless the medicine is to be measured with a pipette or dropper – for example, Nystatin oral suspension. The name of the medicine should be written clearly and not abbreviated.

Directions for the patient will be in English on the label; if you are handwriting a prescription it is still preferable to write it in English but there are some Latin abbreviations which continue to be used. Some of these are shown at the back of the BNF.

There are some slightly different requirements for computer-issued prescriptions which you can see in the BNF online or in the hard copy (BNF, 2022).

Prescriptions for controlled drugs

Changes to the Misuse of Drugs Act (1971, plus amendments) in 2012 meant that nurse and pharmacist independent prescribers were able to prescribe controlled drugs except diamorphine, dipipanone and cocaine for addicts. These controlled drugs can be prescribed for other appropriate uses. Doctors would need a Home Office licence to prescribe these drugs for addicts. For healthcare independent prescribers other than nurses and pharmacists, there are restrictions on which controlled drugs, if any, can be prescribed (Misuse of Drugs (Amendment No.2), 2012).

In Competency 8 of the *Competency Framework for All Prescribers* (RPS, 2021), Prescribe professionally, statement 8.3 states: 'Knows and works within legal and regulatory frameworks'; the further information (b) adds that the 'Frameworks [are] for prescribing controlled drugs, unlicensed and off-label medicines, supplementary prescribing, and prescribing for self, close family and friends'. This section looks at prescribing controlled drugs specifically. There are also sections in this book on licensed and unlicensed medicines and prescribing for close family, self and friends.

What are controlled drugs and what are the classes and schedules?

The Misuse of Drugs Act 1971 divides controlled drugs into three classes, A, B and C, which determine the range of penalties for illegal or unlicensed possession and possession with intent to supply.

For prescriptions, you are more interested in the five schedules which identify the levels of control that the pharmacy makes such as storage and the requirements for the writing of a prescription. **Box 10.1** shows the different schedules with examples of what is in each.

Box 10.1

- Schedule 1 – CDs with no medicinal purposes (e.g., cannabis, LSD)
- Schedule 2 – CDs including opiates (morphine etc.) and major stimulants such as amphetamines
- Schedule 3 – Barbiturates (except quinalbarbitone), and minor stimulants, such as midazolam
- Schedule 4 – Part I Benzodiazepines such as diazepam
- Part II Anabolic/androgenic steroids
- Schedule 5 – CDs with lower risk of abuse (codeine, dihydrocodeine, pholcodine)

The usual prescription requirements described above also apply to prescriptions for controlled drugs; however, there are additional requirements which must be adhered to.

The additional requirements for controlled drug prescriptions

You will not be prescribing schedule 1 drugs but the additional requirements for schedules 2 and 3 are as follows.

The patient's name and address: This is the usual address, but if the patient does not have a fixed address, the words no fixed abode or NFA are acceptable. Use of a post office box is not acceptable.

The signature of the prescriber with the date: In cases such as repeat prescriptions the prescription can be signed by another prescriber other than the named prescriber. However, the address must relate to the signatory of the prescription to be legally valid. The date needs to be the date the prescription was signed. CD prescriptions are valid only for 28 days from the 'appropriate date'. This will usually be the date the prescription was signed but there are exceptions – for example, there may be a date before which the prescription cannot be supplied and it is 28 days from that date. This 28-day rule applies not only to schedules 2 and 3, but also 4 which includes benzodiazepines.

The address of the prescriber: This must be the address of the prescriber and be in the UK.

Name of the controlled drug: It is good practice to write this in full.

The form (capsules, tablets etc.): This must be stated. You can use abbreviations for this. Take care when prescribing modified release (M/R) or sustained release S/R to ensure you make it unambiguous.

The strength: This needs to be written on the prescription, particularly if the medicine is available in more than one strength.

The dose: This must be clearly defined. There are doses that are not legal for a CD prescription and, of course, there are doses that are. **Boxes 10.2** and **10.3** show examples of these.

The total quantity: This must be written in both words and figures. It can be expressed as either the total number of dosage units required or the total quantity of drug in milligrams. For example, 50 (fifty) mg. If the prescription is for a liquid medicine the total quantity should be the volume required.

The quantity prescribed: It is strongly recommended that the maximum quantity for schedules 2, 3 and 4 should not exceed 30 days. This is not a legal restriction but you may be asked to justify any longer period.

Box 10.2 Examples of doses that are not legally acceptable

- As directed
- When required
- PRN
- As per chart
- Titration dose
- Weekly (as this is a frequency and not a dose)
- Twice a day

Box 10.3 Examples of acceptable doses for CDs

- One as directed
- Two when required
- One PRN
- One to two when required

Controlled drugs can be prescribed in instalments, although you may not come across this very often. The details of how to prescribe CDs as instalments is given in the BNF, but is beyond the scope of this short book.

Generic prescribing

An excellent discussion about generic and brand prescribing can be found in Brennan (2022). You will be well aware that we are all expected to prescribe by the generic name of any medicine unless there is a reason for using the brand name. Generic prescribing uses what is called the international non-proprietary name (INN). There are two forms of branded preparation: the proprietary or brand name, or a branded generic name; this can be confusing.

Question 10.1

Why do you think it is important to use generic names when possible? See **Response 10.1** for some suggestions.

Response 10.1

The obvious first answer is generic medicines are generally (although not always) cheaper than the branded proprietary medicine. The Drug Tariff (see Chapter 2) shows the generic reimbursement price the pharmacist will receive when the prescription was written as a generic medicine.

If there are a number of medicines in the same therapeutic area, the brand names may all be very different and not indicate which therapeutic group they belong to. For example, Axid, Pepcid, Tagamet and Ranitidine do not necessarily sound as though they act in a similar way but the generic names of nizatidine, famotidine, cimetidine and ranitidine do show a similarity and they are all H_2 receptor antagonists.

Medicines have only one generic name (the INN), but there may be a number of different 'branded generics' which could be given to the patient who hands in a prescription written for a generic drug. The advantage is that the patient will receive an appropriate medicine, but the disadvantage is that it may cause confusion if the patient receives a different 'branded generic' each time.

However, there are times when it is important that a propriety branded medicine is prescribed rather than a generic one.

Question 10.2

Can you think of any times this may have been discussed? What reasons can you think of? See **Response 10.2** for some examples, but this is not comprehensive.

Response 10.2

Narrow therapeutic index

As discussed in Chapter 6, some drugs have a narrow therapeutic index (the comparison of the amount of a medicine that causes the therapeutic effect to the amount that causes toxicity). This is important, particularly if bioavailability (amount reaching the systemic circulation) differs between the different available 'generic brands'. Examples of drugs with a narrow therapeutic index and where prescribing by brand name would be recommended include: ciclosporin, where patients should be stabilised on a particular brand of oral ciclosporin (switching between formulations without close monitoring may lead to clinically important changes in blood ciclosporin concentration); lithium; certain drugs used for the control of epilepsy such as carbamazepine and phenytoin; and modified-release preparations such as diltiazem, nifedipine and methyl phenidate.

Devices

Some inhalers where the use of a large volume spacer may require a specific brand of inhaler to be effective. Other medicines where a specific device is needed for administration such as adrenaline or insulin.

Opioid patches

For example, buprenorphine transdermal patches are available as 72-hourly, 96-hourly and seven-day formulations. Brand name prescribing is recommended to reduce the risk of confusion and error in dispensing and administration.

Patient adherence

For some patients, differences in product name, presentation, appearance or taste may lead to anxiety, confusion, dosing errors and reduced adherence. If you are about to prescribe a medicine which is likely to be required long term, it is important that you ensure the patient is able to adhere. It is not cost-effective to prescribe a generic medicine that is not taken by the patient.

There are many other medicines where a brand name should be specified. Although a comprehensive list may not be easily obtained, Brennan (2022) is very useful. Also check the SPS list which is updated regularly (SPS, 2023); you may need to register but it is free. Other lists exist and you may wish to contact the ICB or Medicine Committee to see if they have their own lists.

Unlicensed and off-label medicines

In the *Competency Framework for All Prescribers* (RPS, 2021), Competency 4, Prescribe, has two specific statements that refer to this type of prescribing: 4.11: 'Prescribes unlicensed and off-label medicines where legally permitted, and unlicensed medicines only if satisfied that an alternative licensed medicine would not meet the patient's clinical needs' and 4.12: 'Follows appropriate safeguards if prescribing medicines that are unlicensed, off-label, or outside standard practice'.

In order to promote a medicine, a pharmaceutical company must apply for and receive a licence. The licence states the indication(s) for which the medicine can be used; the doses that can be used; how the medicine should be given, for example by mouth, or via injection; and which group of patients it can be used for, such as only adults over 18.

Unlicensed medicine means simply that a licence for this medicine has not been granted but it may still be appropriate to prescribe it. For a definition of unlicensed, see **Box 10.4**.

Box 10.4

Unlicensed refers to medicines that are not licensed for any indication or age group because the drug:

- is undergoing a clinical trial or
- has been imported or
- has been prepared extemporaneously or
- was prepared under a special manufacturing licence.

Most trusts will have a policy for dealing with unlicensed medicines. As a nurse prescriber you are allowed to prescribe unlicensed medicines if no licensed medicine is available, but you must be satisfied that an alternative, licensed medicine would not meet the patient's needs.

You must be satisfied that there is a sufficient evidence base or experience of use to demonstrate the medicine's safety and efficacy for your patient and, very importantly, you must inform the patient and they must agree to a prescription in the knowledge that the drug is unlicensed; they must understand the implications of this. Finally, the medicine chosen and the reason for choosing it should be documented in the patient's notes.

Off-label medicines

There will be times when the medicine you are to prescribe is called off-label. This means it is a licensed medicine but is being used for an unlicensed condition or outside the terms of its licence in some other way.

There are a number of circumstances in which you can prescribe licensed medicines for the purposes for which they are not licensed (this is most likely to be the case when prescribing for children). However, in order to do so the prescriber must ensure the following conditions are met.

- You must be satisfied that it would better serve the patient's needs than an appropriately licensed alternative.
- You must be satisfied that there is a sufficient evidence base and/or experience for using the medicine to demonstrate its safety and efficacy.
- You must explain to the patient, or parent/carer, in broad terms, the reasons why medicines are not licensed for their proposed use.
- You must keep a clear, accurate and legible record of all medicines prescribed and the reasons for prescribing an 'off-label' medicine.
- Examples are shown in Box 10.5.

Box 10.5 Examples of off-label use

- Use of a licensed medicine for an age group that is not included in its licence – for example, a medicine licensed for adults but being used for children.
- Use of a licensed medicine for an illness that is not included in its licence.
- Use of a medicine that is only available from abroad and has to be imported (it may have a licence in other countries).
- Use of a medicine that needs to be made specially because it cannot be obtained easily – for example, a patient may not be able to swallow a tablet or capsule (which is licensed) and needs a liquid (unlicensed) version of the medicine.

Many medicines that are widely given to children are used in a way that is unlicensed. This gives you more choice about which medicine to use than if they could only use licensed medicines.

Most medicines are not licensed for use in pregnant women but it may be essential that they are used (see Chapter 8). Have a look at the BNF and see if you can note down some of the unlicensed uses of licensed medicines. See **Box 10.6** for some examples of medicines in the BNF that have restrictions to the licence.

Box 10.6 Examples of licensed medicines used in an unlicensed way

- Sumatriptan is not licensed for use in the elderly.
- Atenolol is not licensed for use in migraine prophylaxis.
- Ibuprofen is not licensed for children under three months.

- Methotrexate is not licensed for use in severe Crohn's disease.
- Domperidone is no longer indicated for the relief of nausea and vomiting in children aged under 12 years or those weighing less than 35kg.
- Salmeterol is not licensed for children under the age of 12.
- Capsaicin is used in the treatment of localised neuropathic pain but is not licensed for this indication.
- Cyclizine tablets are not licensed for use in children under six years. The injection is not licensed for use in children of any age.
- Naproxen is used for the treatment of acute migraine in combination with sumatriptan but is not licensed for this indication.
- Senna tablets are not licensed for use in children under six years. Senna syrup is not licensed for use in children under two years.

There are many more, so always check the BNF if you are not sure. Most of these restrictions relate to the age of the patient or their medical condition.

As well as following the guidelines above for prescribing for patients face to face, we need to consider how we deal with patients when we are contacting them remotely such as on the telephone.

Risks associated with remote prescribing

What is remote prescribing?

Remote prescribing is prescribing that occurs in the context of the prescriber and the patient being physically or geographically remote from each other (Broadhead, 2020) and can include situations where a prescription is generated during a telephone or internet-based consultation. Remote prescribing may also take place by email, fax, or website.

The *Competency Framework for All Prescribers* (RPS, 2021) has a number of competencies and supporting statements which relate to safe prescribing and minimising risk. One in particular relates to remote prescribing. Competency 7, Prescribe safely, has the supporting statements 7.3: 'Identifies and minimises potential risks associated with prescribing via remote methods' and 7.4: 'Recognises when safe prescribing processes are not in place and acts to minimise risks'.

Over the last decade there have been significant increases in the number of consultations undertaken remotely using supportive digital health technologies. Why do you think this is?

It is due to multiple factors including significant innovations in technology that have led to the development of more effective tele-health platforms. As these technologies have become more accessible and usable in a healthcare setting this has led to changes in models of care provision. This means that not only telephone communication can be undertaken, but also virtual consultations using video links and real-time conversations.

The COVID-19 global pandemic (which began in 2020) significantly increased the use of remote health platforms; during that time you will have noticed an increase in the number of consultations being undertaken remotely as a response to the emerging pandemic and to the implementation of national lockdowns in the UK and across the globe (Patel et al., 2021).

Currently, the UK is no longer working under COVID-19 restrictions, but is it highly likely that many prescribers will remain involved in the delivery of care using remote consultation. Indeed, the increasing implementation of digital technologies to support care provision and empower patients is a strategic aim of England's *NHS Long Term Plan* (NHS England, 2019), Scotland's *Digital Health and Care Strategy* (Scottish Government, 2018) and Wales's *A Healthier Wales: Long Term Plan for Health and Social Care* (Welsh Government, 2018). The use of digital healthcare in the future is likely to increase, resulting in increasing numbers of prescribers involved in remote prescribing in order to meet the commitment to support patients with better control of their care. What do you think patients think of this?

What does this mean for you as a prescriber?

For primary care practitioners this might mean an increase in consultations undertaken by telephone or video link. Secondary care practitioners might experience remote prescribing differently, with technologies permitting follow-up and prescribing away from the bedside and in clinical facilities distant from the patient.

Remote prescribing is risky

As a prescriber, you need to embed these safe practices. The risky nature of this prescribing activity is something that the regulatory bodies are very aware of.

In the *Competency Framework for All Prescribers* (RPS, 2021), Competency 7 Prescribe safely, has the supporting statement 7.3: 'Identifies and minimises potential risks associated with prescribing via remote methods with further information being remote methods include telephone, email, video or communication via a third party'.

The Care Quality Commission (CQC) acknowledges that well-run remote services can offer patients a convenient, safe and effective alternative to face-to-face healthcare but warns of risks inherent in the system that might not be appropriately assessed or managed (CQC, 2017 updated 2022). The professional regulatory bodies have responded to this with the provision of guidance in relation to remote prescribing. This guidance from the NMC, the GMC and the General Pharmaceutical Council (GPhC) is welcome and of use to all prescribers who might be required to undertake remote consultation and prescribing. See the remote prescribing high-level principles below.

The areas of risk that tend to be highlighted include concerns that during online consultations there are challenges confirming the true identity of the patient and that issues with a person's capacity can be difficult to fully evaluate. It has been identified that inadequate medication history-taking is a risk and that there can be barriers to adequate follow-up for monitoring, especially if a consultation is undertaken by a practitioner different to the original prescriber (CQC, 2017 updated 2022).

How to develop safe practice in remote consultation and prescribing

Remote consultations and prescribing are here to stay and are likely to increase with greater pressure put on face-to-face appointments and potentially patient preference gained over the years of the pandemic. As a nurse prescriber you will be at the forefront driving its success and in mitigating the potential risks associated. Remember that prescribing needs to be patient-centred; remote prescribing will have an important place but it should not become the norm. Face-to-face consultations need to be the mainstay of the prescribing and consultation process (see Chapter 3).

It is essential for you as a nurse prescriber to develop your practice to put the safety of the patient at the forefront. Broadhead (2020) notes that the success is dependent on prescribers developing robust consultation techniques, strengthening approaches to gaining valid consent, building effective dialogue, fostering rapport, accurate history-taking and observation of the patient when required. Chapter 3 discusses this in more detail.

You have a responsibility to assess the situation to evaluate whether you are able to prescribe safely when acting remotely. Prescribing safely requires a confidence in knowledge about the patient's health and an understanding that this remote encounter can safely meet the patient's needs. You should undertake a risk–benefit analysis to ensure that this approach enhances effective treatment and will not expose the patient to increased harm (Broadhead, 2020).

You need to be confident to be able to assess the patient and offer face-to-face appointments if any issues arise during the remote consultation. Red flags that should prompt a deeper weighing up of the risks and benefits should include: consultations with patients with complex care needs; where high-risk treatments are likely to be prescribed; and consultations where it is uncertain if the person has capacity. Limited access to patient records should also prompt a deeper consideration of the appropriateness of a remote consultation potentially leading to a prescribing opportunity, especially if the patient is typically under the care of another practitioner.

You should also ensure you assess the IT infrastructure in use in the clinical area in which you practice and evaluate whether it is a barrier to effective communication. The patient's access to dependable technology and internet is also imperative. In the event of a poor-quality internet connection or phone line then arranging a face-to-face consultation will be more appropriate as it aids communication and information provision (Greenhalgh et al., 2021).

To provide patients with effective safeguards, the UK health regulatory bodies have co-authored high-level principles for remote prescribing. The principles are for all healthcare professionals with prescribing responsibilities. The list of co-authors is shown in **Box 10.7**. They are summarised in **Box 10.8**; you should use them to govern your practice as a prescribing nurse (GMC, 2022).

Box 10.7 Co-authors of the principles

- Academy of Medical Royal Colleges
- Care Quality Commission
- Faculty of Pain Medicine
- General Dental Council
- General Medical Council
- General Pharmaceutical Council
- Healthcare Improvement Scotland
- Healthcare Inspectorate Wales

- Nursing and Midwifery Council
- Pharmaceutical Society of Northern Ireland
- Regulation and Quality improvement Authority
- Royal Pharmaceutical Society

Box 10.8 Remote prescribing high-level principles

Co-authored and agreed by several regulators, Royal colleges and healthcare bodies, including the NMC; reproduced with kind permission.

Principle 1

Make patient safety the first priority and raise concerns if the service or system you are working in does not have adequate patient safeguards, including appropriate identity and verification checks.

Principle 2

Understand how to identify vulnerable patients and take appropriate steps to protect them.

Principle 3

Tell patients your name, role, and (if online) professional registration details, establish a dialogue and make sure the patient understands how the remote consultation is going to work.

Principle 4

Explain that:

a. they can only prescribe if it is safe to do so.
b. it's not safe if they don't have sufficient information about the patient's health or if remote care is unsuitable to meet their needs.
c. it may be unsafe if relevant information is not shared with other healthcare providers involved in their care.
d. if they can't prescribe because it's unsafe they will signpost to other appropriate services.

Principle 5

Obtain informed consent and follow relevant mental capacity law and codes of practice.

Principle 6

Undertake an adequate clinical assessment and access medical records or verify important information by examination or testing where necessary.

Principle 7

Give patients information about all the options available to them, including declining treatment, in a way they can understand.

Principle 8

Make appropriate arrangements for after care and, unless the patient objects, share all relevant information with colleagues and other health and social care providers involved in their care to support ongoing monitoring and treatment.

Principle 9

Keep notes that fully explain and justify the decisions they make.

Principle 10

Stay up to date with relevant training, support and guidance for providing healthcare in a remote context.

Developing the quality of your remote consultation is key

When remote prescribing is linked to a remote consultation you need to develop safe strategies for the consultation and keep in mind the fundamental aspects of accountability and responsibility (Shepherd, 2019). You should also be aware of barriers that can inhibit safety – for example, Greenhalgh et al. identify the risk of patients downplaying symptoms on e-consultations to avoid an algorithm-driven diversion to a call-handling service (2021). Consideration also needs to be given to patients with additional communication needs. In some situations, an online consultation might be preferable, but some people may need additional digital access support to fully engage in remote consultations. Younger people might be more able to access remote consultations in comparison to the older population and this might need to be addressed in some way to ensure equity of access (Patel et al., 2021).

Issues such as confidentiality and privacy should be explored, especially for vulnerable patients who might be at risk from eavesdropping. Safeguarding principles should be applied to all remote consultations and you, as the prescriber, should be aware and take reasonable steps to optimise confidentiality and privacy (Shepherd, 2019).

There is also some emerging evidence that remote consultations may impact upon typical professional relationships. Greenhalgh et al. (2021, p. 4) describe 'The unfamiliarity and strangeness of communication via video, including some people's dislike of seeing their own face or body on video and a sense of inappropriate intimacy (e.g., a doctor's discomfort at seeing a patient part-naked in a bedroom rather than on an examination couch)'. You need to take this into account and adapt your consultation skills as required.

While it is not always ideal for a prescriber to make prescribing decisions while physically absent from the patient, it is likely this approach to healthcare will increase with the increasing reliance on digital technologies. In some cases, remote prescribing will improve patient care and enhance patient control and self-management of their condition.

The NMC (2022) stipulates that you must prescribe in line with the requirements of *The Code* and your individual scope of practice, so it is important for you as a nurse prescriber to be aware of the potential risks associated with remote prescribing. As well as the immediate risks to the safety of individual patients, structural and economic issues such as digital exclusion and low digital literacy need some consideration.

Remember the remote prescribing high-level principles and be aware that you are responsible for every prescription you sign. When engaging in remote prescribing it is essential that patient safety is a priority.

Summary

This chapter concentrated on prescription writing, including a discussion about prescribing of licensed, unlicensed or off-label medicines and prescribing controlled drugs.

It considered when generic prescribing is appropriate and when it is not.

Finally, it discussed the risks associated with prescribing via remote methods such as the telephone. It reproduces the co-authored and agreed ten high-level principles which are for all healthcare professionals with prescribing responsibilities when prescribing remotely.

References

BNF 2022. *British National Formulary: Key Information on the Selection, Prescribing, Dispensing and Administration of Medicines.* Available at bnf.nice.org.uk/ (accessed December 2022).

Brennan, K. 2022. *Prescribing by Generic or Brand Name in Primary Care.* Specialist Pharmacy Services. Available at www.sps.nhs.uk/articles/prescribing-by-generic-or-brand-name-in-primary-care/#:~:text=generic%20prescribing (accessed 31 May 2023).

Broadhead, R. 2020. Remote prescribing. *Journal of Prescribing Practice.* **2**, pp. 380–2.

CQC 2019. *Online Primary Care: Response from the Regulators.* Available at www.cqc.org.uk/news/stories/online-primary-care-response-regulators (accessed 13 July 2022).

CQC 2017 (updated 2022). *Care Quality Commission Advises People to Take Care When Using Online Primary Care Services.* Available at www.cqc.org.uk/news/releases/care-quality-commission-advises-people-take-care-when-using-online-primary-care (accessed 13 July 2023).

EL 2018. (91) 127 *Responsibility for Prescribing Between Hospitals and GPs.* Superseded by NHS England, 2018.

General Medical Council (GMC) 2021. *Remote Consultations.* Available at www.gmc-uk.org/ethical-guidance/ethical-hub/remote-consultations (accessed 13 July 2022).

GMC 2022. *Remote Prescribing High Level Principles.* Available at www.gmc-uk.org/ethical-guidance/learning-materials/remote-prescribing-high-level-principles (accessed 13 July 2022).

Greenhalgh, T., Rosen, R., Shaw, S.E., Byng, R., Faulkner, S., Finlay, T., Grundy, E., Husain, L., Hughes, G., Leone, C., Moore, L., Papoutsi, C., Pope, C., Rybczynska-Bunt, S., Rushforth, A., Wherton, J., Wieringa, S. and Wood, G.W. 2021. *Planning and Evaluating Remote Consultation Services: A New Conceptual Framework Incorporating Complexity and Practical Ethics. Frontiers in Digital Health* (3) Available at www.frontiersin.org/articles/10.3389/fdgth.2021.726095 (accessed 31 May 2023).

Misuse of Drugs Act 1971. Available at www.legislation.gov.uk/ukpga/1971/38/contents (accessed 31 May 2023).

Misuse of Drugs (Amendment No. 2) 2012. Statutory instrument 973. Available at www.legislation.gov.uk/uksi/2012/973/made (accessed December 2022).

NHS England 2018. *Responsibility for Prescribing Between Primary and Secondary/Tertiary Care.* Available at www.england.nhs.uk/wp-content/uploads/2018/03/responsibility-prescribing-between-primary-secondary-care-v2.pdf (accessed December 2022).

NHS England 2019. *The NHS Long Term Plan.* Available at: www.longtermplan.nhs.uk/wp-content/uploads/2019/08/nhs-long-term-plan-version-1.2.pdf (accessed 26 September 2022).

Nursing and Midwifery Council (NMC) 2022. *Useful Information for Prescribers.* Available at www.nmc.org.uk/standards/standards-for-post-registration/standards-for-prescribers/useful-information-for-prescribers/ (accessed 13 July 2022).

Patel, R., Irving, J., Brinn, A., Broadbent, M., Shetty, H., Pritchard, M., Downs, J., Stewart, R., Harland, R. and McGuire, P. 2021. Impact of the COVID-19 pandemic on remote mental healthcare and prescribing in psychiatry: An electronic health record study. *BMJ Open.* **11**, e046365.

RPS 2021. *A Competency Framework for All Prescribers.* Available at www.rpharms.com/resources/frameworks/prescribing-competency-framework/competency-framework (accessed 12 May 2023).

Scottish Government 2018. *Digital Health and Care Strategy.* Available at https://www.gov.scot/publications/scotlands-digital-health-care-strategy/#:~:text=In%202018%2C%20Scotland's%20first%20Digital,the%20use%20of%20digital%20technology (accessed 21 September 2023).

Shepherd, A.B. 2019. To prescribe or not to prescribe: Enhancing safety in remote prescribing. *Journal of Prescribing Practice.* **1**(3), pp. 139–44.

SPS 2023. *Example Medicines to Prescribe by Brand Name in Primary Care.* Available at www.sps.nhs.uk/articles/example-medicines-to-prescribe-by-brand-name-in-primary-care/ (accessed April 2023).

Welsh Government 2018. *A Healthier Wales: Long Term Plan for Health and Social Care.* Available at https://www.gov.wales/healthier-wales-long-term-plan-health-and-social-care (accessed 21 September 2023).

11

Transition to Prescriber and Deprescribing

Lorraine Henshaw, Barry Strickland-Hodge
and Daniel Okeowo

Chapter summary

This chapter draws on recent research looking at:

- the transition from qualified nurse to prescriber;
- the need for continuing professional development;
- deprescribing.

Transition to nurse prescriber

Your role as a prescriber is likely to be very different to your role as a nurse. If you have already qualified as a prescriber, you may smile to think of the change. In Chapter 4, we discussed team working and the need for a multidisciplinary approach to your role as prescriber. In the *Competency Framework for All Prescribers* (RPS, 2021), Competency 10 is Prescribe as part of a team; this is very important, particularly when you are newly qualified as a prescriber. The supporting statements for Competency 10 all discuss the need not to be isolated in your new role and to ask for support when you need it. In fact, they suggest you agree an appropriate level of support from the outset. This short section looks at the transition from qualified nurse, where you may have worked in a team, to nurse prescriber. Make sure you understand the issues around this transition where your decisions on what to prescribe will have an important influence on the health of your patient.

This transition happens more frequently than you may think. You may not immediately agree, but transition is a concept that affects all of us, throughout our lives, at many different stages and in many ways – for example, moving from one school year to another, moving house, becoming a parent, moving jobs and even a shift in health status, such as the diagnosis of a long-term condition. This underlines how transition is the key to many of the significant events in our lives. Maybe because of this, a range of theories have been developed to offer an explanation of the concept of transition, both in a general sense, such as transitions that can happen to everyone (Van Gennep, 1960; Bridges, 2004), and in more focused subject area-specific fields, such as the move from student nurse to becoming a qualified nurse (Benner, 1984; Duchscher, 2008; Kramer, 1974; Wray et al., 2021).

The different transition theories and related research literature discuss transition as being a process through which we have to go to transform or reach an end point, encompassing a change (Kralik et al., 2006). One of the most often cited general theorists, Bridges (2004), characterises transition as a linear process, or a series of steps. He describes three stages during a transition: an ending, a neutral zone and a new beginning, claiming all transitions must start with an ending, where the individual must leave something behind – for example, moving job or changing status in that job – and that transitions conclude with a fresh beginning, as we emerge into the new state, whatever that may be. The neutral zone is the 'in-betweenness', a stage sandwiched between the then and the now or the ending and the new beginning. Other theories, such as those by Fisher (2008) and Van Gennep (1960), are similar, with movement through phases until a new state; however, other theories claim this is not simply linear but more dynamic in nature (Kralik et al., 2006). There is some agreement in these theories, however, that whatever the mechanism of transition, the transition period itself can be difficult, with many challenges (Kralik et al., 2006).

Let's consider the transitions you have faced so far in your personal and professional lives for a minute. Think about the processes and reflect upon the experiences for a while, if you will. How did you feel?

Within your move from qualified nurse to nurse prescriber, you may experience some or all of the known challenges of transition to some degree or another; by discussing some of the key points of this here we hope to be able to provide you with some understanding of what you may be experiencing and what steps can be taken to smooth the process.

There is, for example, a whole raft of evidence surrounding transition in a health professional context, most notably within nursing, where the process of transition from student to newly qualified nurse (NQN) has been the focus. You may be aware of some of this work, particularly in your role in practice learning environments as a practice assessor or supervisor, supporting student nurses, or it may be something new to you; either way, it is worth considering this here.

Much of this research (Benner, 1984; Kramer, 1974; Duchsher, 2008, 2009; Wray et al., 2021) highlights important factors for successful transition to NQN, including previous experience, skills acquisition and mastery, and the support and acceptance of others in the healthcare team. The research also identifies many of the problems NQNs face during this transition period, including things like managing expectations of self and others, lack of self-reliance and confidence, managing complex workloads, fitting in, teamwork and apprehension about ability and performance (Joseph et al., 2022).

There are lots of reasons for difficulties during transition to the NQN, but included in these is the mismatch of expectations as a student nurse leaves behind the protection of the student status for the responsibility and accountability of the NQN. You may have experienced this for yourself in one respect or another and understand that how support is offered at this time is fundamental to be success of this huge milestone.

Research has also looked at the transition from one healthcare professional role to another and this highlights issues with identity and autonomy as additional important concepts. In fact, recent research by Henshaw (2021) has concluded that transition from an established role, such as your current position as a qualified nurse, is influenced by a range of factors including challenges to role identity, adapting to new ways of working, accessing support during transition and acceptance within the new role.

Let's first look at identity and consider how this can be impacted by moving into a new role. The motivation to become a nurse is linked very much to how we want to help others, to be altruistic, seeing it as a vocation; on the whole, we tend to consider ourselves not as just 'doing' nursing but we actually have a strong connection to 'being' a nurse. We develop a firm allegiance to the profession, seeing it not just as a role but part of who we are. Any changes to this, even those that may enhance the role, can be experienced as a threat, developing a sense of vulnerability and a strong urge to protect what is known, familiar and safe – that is, your identity as a nurse.

In your transition to a nurse prescriber role you will likely experience changes to this sense of identity as you move into the prescribing role and as you adjust to the new sense of self it will bring. As well as how you see yourself, becoming a nurse prescriber will undoubtably cause you to be looked at differently by others, adding to the tension around your identity. So don't be surprised if this causes some anxiety and stress, especially as you adapt and learn to manage the identities of nurse and nurse prescriber together. In the research by Henshaw (2021) the participants learned to balance their multiple identities through a process of trial and error, moving between the identities as they grew in confidence or reverting back to the original identity if they became overly stressed, helping them to feel safe again until they were ready to move on towards the newer identity. You may also experiment with your new role as a prescriber, going back and forth between nurse and nurse prescriber while you are in the transition period until you feel confident and accepted in this new reframed you.

You will obviously also be changing the way you work and interact with patients as you take on your prescribing role and attain heightened autonomy and responsibility for assessment and prescribing (albeit within your scope of practice). You may, however, lack confidence and competencies as you move from what you knew well in your established qualified nurse role to that of a nurse prescriber, feeling the mismatch between your previous skills and expertise and the newly required knowledge and proficiencies that will allow you to prescribe safely, maintaining the quality of patient care. These changes may impact on your self-esteem and wellbeing. You are, in a sense, having to relinquish some of the autonomy you had in your previous non-prescribing role, where you felt at ease and comfortable making decisions in practice, decisions based on your clinical expertise in your role at the time. For some this shift in autonomy may lead to a real sense of loss and reduced confidence for a while, which could be perceived as a threat to self-worth. In my research this loss was even compared to grief by some participants. However, as the new role becomes more familiar through support, practice and increasing competence this improves – eventually culminating in a regaining of confidence and a rebuilding of competencies, now appropriate to your role as a nurse prescriber. Actually, support and acceptance in the new role are vital to a successful transition and the environment, the team and the wider peers that you work with will be really important here. There has been some important research by Wenger (1998, 2010) establishing that acceptance from peers is vital in helping people to become part of a new group. Her research identified the concept of a community of practice which is basically a network or a group of like-minded peers. The important thing about this is sharing of certain attributes such as a language, values, knowledge base, history and tools. It is this sharing that provides a support network and a sense of belonging, providing strength and resources to its members. A community of practice (CoP) can relate to anything, but it will have all the characteristics mentioned above. So, a CoP of a nursing speciality, for example, shares the same language (in terms of phrases and meanings – that is, 'cares' for neonatal nursing), the same education, the same values, the same tools. As a nurse prescriber who is part of a CoP of nurse prescribers, there will be different language (i.e., around prescribing), different education, different tools etc. shared to those outside the CoP.

The tricky thing here can be that it is not always easy, first, to leave behind an existing CoP and, second, to get acceptance to join a new CoP. This is because the move away from the existing one brings with it the sense of loss, as already discussed, causing anxiety and a sense of vulnerability; joining a new one relies on its existing members allowing you in. One thing you can do to help is to seek support from the new CoP current members, to build ties with this group. So, for you the existing nurse prescribing community and your assessors and supervisor will be important as you manage this transition. In my research acceptance into these new groups was also affected by the way clients/patients and other members of the MDT saw the participants.

Having the ability to prescribe will fundamentally change the way you approach your caregiving and increase your level of autonomy, but all this takes time to adjust to; you may find this period stressful and feel the impact on your wellbeing. One way to support your transition to a nurse prescriber role is by ensuring you engage with continuing professional development.

Continuing professional development

In the introduction to the *Competency Framework for All Prescribers* (RPS, 2021), it mentions continuing professional development (CPD) and how the framework can be used to guide this.

It can be used to help healthcare professionals prepare to prescribe and provide the basis for ongoing continuing education and development programmes, as well as revalidation processes. For example, it can be used as a framework for a portfolio to demonstrate continued competency in prescribing.

The NMC *Standards of Proficiency* state: 'Our standards of proficiency can be a key resource when planning CPD as part of your revalidation' (2018b). In Competency 9 of the *Framework* (RPS, 2021), Improve professional practice, two of the supporting statements are: 9.4 'Takes responsibility for own learning and continuing professional development relevant to the prescribing role' and 9.6: 'Encourages and supports others with their prescribing practice and continuing professional development'. In the further information that follows, it adds that these aims can be achieved: c. 'By continuously reviewing, reflecting, identifying gaps, planning, acting, applying and evidencing learning or competencies' and d. 'By considering mentoring, leadership and workforce development (for example, becoming a Designated Prescribing Practitioner)'.

So, the *Competency Framework for All Prescribers* (RPS, 2021) can become the centre of CPD.

What is CPD and what is the difference between that and continuing education?

Continuing education is a largely passive activity, such as attendance at conferences and courses, whereas CPD is an active process which involves not just attending a training event, but also a reflection as to how this might change your practice. It is a cyclical process of reflection on practice, planning, action and evaluation (reflection on learning) (see **Box 11.1**).

Box 11.1

A Chief Medical Officer's report from 1998 (CMO, 1998) stated that the core principles of CPD were:

- purposeful and patient-centred;
- participative, involving the individual and other stakeholders;
- targeted at identified educational need;
- educationally effective;
- part of a wider organisational development plan in support of local and national service objectives;
- focused on development needs of clinical teams across traditional professional boundaries;
- designed to build on previous knowledge, skills and experience;
- designed to enhance the skills of interpreting and applying knowledge based on research and development.

CPD includes everything that you learn which makes you better able to do your job. All definitions of CPD try to describe an educational system which seeks to operate throughout your working life, mirrors the requirements imposed upon you by your professional bodies and, equally important, your patients. It should also operate in a systematic and structured manner and cover the full range of knowledge and skills – personal, technical and commercial – required by you as a professional in your working life.

CPD could be defined as the process through which healthcare professionals continuously enhance their knowledge, skills and personal qualities throughout their professional careers. It is generally considered to be a four-stage cycle:

*   identifying training needs (reflection);
*   deciding how to meet these training needs (planning);
*   taking part in training activities (action);
*   evaluating performance (evaluation).

To be effective, CPD must be an integral part of your organisation's strategy. It should be considered as an investment in the total skill base of the workforce and organisations should ensure that MDTs learn together (see Chapter 4). It is intended to increase learning, not just to offer training in specific skills. To be effective, it should be assessed and evaluated in order to measure effectiveness and be applicable to different staff members and flexible enough to reflect their requirements. Overall, it can be a catalyst for change in the workplace.

Therefore, it should be a partnership between the individual and the organisation; time should be made available. If you do not grasp a self-directed approach to CPD there is a danger that organisations may develop a purely risk-management process for ensuring CPD. CPD seeks to establish a GOAL.

Gaps in current levels of professional competence.

Opportunities for career development and additional skills required.

Aims and objectives of the CPD process for the individual.

Learning from an evaluation of CPD activities to date.

What is the importance of CPD? See **Box 11.2** for some ideas.

Box 11.2

Quality assurance

Requires that adequately trained staff perform all significant roles within an organisation and that the training is kept up to date. Lessons learned in university have a decreasing life span. Roles also change. New skills have to be acquired for career development.

Patients

Increasingly demanding, better informed. Duty of care is a prime responsibility.

The law

Ignorance is no defence and may be seen as an offence! Insurance policies may demand CPD.

> ## Professional standards
>
> Standards of competence require recording of CPD to retain membership.

It should not be seen as gathering points but as improving performance. How can you engage in CPD? What types of CPD are there that could support you? **Box 11.3** has some suggestions.

> ## Box 11.3
>
> - Distance or open learning
> - MDT meetings and learning
> - Case-based discussions with colleagues
> - Structured reading
> - Writing technical papers
> - Membership of relevant professional committees
> - Part-time teaching

The Code: Professional Standards of Practice and Behaviour for Nurses, Midwives and Nursing Associates, originally published by the NMC in 2015 and updated to reflect the regulation of nursing associates in 2018, states:

> 22.2 keep to our prescribed hours of practice and carry out continuing professional development activities
>
> 22.3 keep your knowledge and skills up to date, taking part in appropriate and regular learning and professional development activities that aim to maintain and develop your competence and improve your performance.

(NMC, 2018a)

It is your responsibility to remain up to date with the knowledge and skills to enable you to prescribe competently and safely within your area of expertise. A commitment to CPD throughout your working life is essential in this context and this should encourage all professionals to produce their own CPD plans to indicate their personal and professional goals.

Deprescribing

The emphasis in this short book has been, not surprisingly, on prescribing. It's about how, what and why to prescribe and considers what may appear to be a number of disparate issues and concepts. However, this section is almost the opposite and potentially the most difficult for you as a nurse prescriber. Deprescribing is expected to be taken very seriously by all prescribers, but the need to involve the patient or carer is emphasised again. Think about the potential problems associated with the concept of deprescribing and think about how you might be able to overcome them. The idea behind deprescribing is simple: stop medicines when they are no longer needed in the context of a patient and their treatment goals. However, the term 'deprescribing' was used first in 2003 but has only recently gained more attention from academics, clinicians and policy-makers to reduce 'problematic polypharmacy' (Woodward, 2003).

In the Glossary of the *Competency Framework for All Prescribers* (RPS, 2021, p. 21), deprescribing is defined as:

> The process of stopping or reducing medicines with the aim of eliminating problematic (inappropriate) polypharmacy, and then monitoring the individual for unintended adverse effects or worsening of disease. It is essential to involve the individual (and their carer) closely in deprescribing decisions to build and maintain their confidence in the process.

Furthermore, Competency 2, Identify evidence-based treatment options available for clinical decision making, has supporting statement 2.2: 'Considers all pharmacological treatment options including optimising doses as well as stopping treatment (appropriate polypharmacy and deprescribing)'. In Competency 9, Improve prescribing practice, further information e. states: 'Methods of reducing a medicine's carbon footprint and environmental impact include proper disposal of medicine/device/equipment waste, recycling schemes, avoiding overprescribing and waste through regular reviews, deprescribing, dose and device optimisation'.

The use of medicines continues to increase, making polypharmacy more prevalent in our healthcare system. This is not inherently negative as patients can benefit from taking multiple medicines to combat comorbidities. However, if we do not take time to ensure the necessity of every medicine a patient is taking and don't stop medicines patients no longer need, polypharmacy can quickly become problematic – for example, where multiple medicines have been prescribed inappropriately or where the intended benefit of the medicine is not realised (Duerden et al., 2013). This leads to the negative consequences that we typically attach to polypharmacy, such as an increased risk of ADRs (Pirmohamed et al., 2004). In the short time you have with each patient you may try to ensure any new symptoms are alleviated. You might consider the symptom as an adverse reaction to a drug the patient is already taking, so stopping the first or at least considering whether it should be changed is important.

An intervention you can utilise to reduce 'problematic polypharmacy' is deprescribing. A more succinct definition of deprescribing is: '[A] systematic process of identifying and discontinuing drugs where harms outweigh benefits within the context of an individual patient's care goals, and their current level of functioning' (Scott et al., 2015, p. 827).

There has always been an issue of repeat prescribing continuing long after conditions have improved or where medicines are no longer required. This is not to say that the practice of stopping a medicine has only just been discovered, though much of the deprescribing we currently see in practice is reactive. This means we tend to stop a medicine once there already is a clear clinical or situational trigger, such as newly developed adverse reactions because of that medicine. There is a need for more proactive deprescribing that looks to deprescribe problematic medicines before patient safety is compromised (Anderson et al., 2017). We realise that in a busy healthcare setting there is limited time to consider all the repeat medicines a patient is taking. It may be simpler to re-prescribe them when requested by the patient. However, it is important to remember that deprescribing considers the patient's own care goals, and so shared decision-making is pivotal to making deprescribing work. Deprescribing is not about denying patients medicines but is an agreement between patients and clinicians that is continually monitored. When patients are involved in such decisions, they are better informed about potential outcomes which facilitates better deprescribing (Jansen et al., 2016).

Growing evidence has highlighted how deprescribing is effective in stopping unnecessary medicines. A systematic review of deprescribing trials (also described as medicine withdrawal trials) found evidence for the effectiveness and lack of significant harm when, for example, benzodiazepines were deprescribed (Iyer et al., 2008). Since this, more evidence has continued to be published highlighting how deprescribing can be feasible and lead to important benefits, especially for older people living with frailty (Ibrahim et al., 2021). With such a growing evidence base, one would assume that all prescribers wouldn't hesitate to incorporate deprescribing into their workflow. However, enacting deprescribing comes with its own hurdles and challenges.

Think about the situation when you are in a consultation with a patient who is currently taking a number of medicines. Is this the right time to discuss reducing changing or stopping medicines? Does the patient have any new symptoms that could be side-effects to their existing medicines? Would you prefer to make a plan in advance of the consultation? There have been various methods of involving patients in reducing their potential dependence on benzodiazepine – for example, sending a letter to patients who have been taking these medicines for a long period of time. The letter might first explain why this is important to the patient and suggest simply reducing doses very gradually. Similarly, the letter might ask the patient to contact the practice to talk with you or a colleague, but only if the patient wants to do this. Those that wish to deprescribe will then be in a positive frame of mind and willing to discuss it.

You will, by now, realise that there are many potential barriers stopping a prescriber from initiating a deprescribing process – not only for you, as the healthcare professional, but also for the patient.

Activity 11.1

List the barriers you can think of and check this with Response 11.1. You may have thought of others but these are the ones typically quoted.

Response 11.1

Potential barriers to deprescribing:

- a strong 'pill for every ill' prescribing culture;
- fear of the effects of deprescribing;
- patient attachment to their medicines;
- lack of time to initiate and monitor deprescribing;
- lack of guidance for healthcare professionals on how to deprescribe;
- lack of tools and resources to support deprescribing;
- clinical guidelines rarely account for patients with multiple diseases;
- fragmentation of care;
- you may not be the person who prescribed the medicine initially.

> ### Box 11.4 Potential barriers to deprescribing
>
> Think about seeing a patient for the first time. You have checked their medical notes and you see there are many medicines. Would it matter if you weren't the prescriber who initiated the existing list of drugs to this patient?

Patients may fear the consequences of deprescribing, such as withdrawal effects or return/worsening of the underlying condition or may question the appropriateness of deprescribing (Reeve et al., 2013). Patients may also be reluctant to stop a medicine if it was originally prescribed by a specialist (Linsky et al., 2019). In addition, current overprescribing cultures can encourage patients to expect 'a pill for every ill', therefore leading to further disagreement regarding the idea of stopping medicines (Doherty et al., 2020). That said, it is important to note that research has shown patients would be open to stopping one or more medicines if their prescriber said that they could (Reeve et al., 2013). Educating patients on their medicine indication and the potential risks of its continued use can be useful in helping patients to think about the necessity of their medicines and potentially initiate deprescribing conversations (Ailabouni et al., 2022). This goes hand in hand with research particularly focused on potential harms of the long-term use of medicines, reporting an increased rate of deprescribing as a result (Kuntz et al., 2019; Martin et al., 2018).

For you, as a healthcare professional and prescriber, key deprescribing hurdles are shown in **Response 11.1**. Prescribers have described deprescribing as time-consuming compared to prescribing, which is perceived as the easier option and adds to the overprescribing culture (Wallis et al., 2017). Are you nodding your head in agreement with this?

A lack of deprescribing resources and guidelines has also been seen to hinder professionals when they need to make deprescribing decisions. This then has a knock-on effect on the prescriber's belief and confidence in being able to enact deprescribing safely (Anderson et al., 2014). Thankfully, increasing research has aided the development of deprescribing tools with more guidelines and resources available for prescribers (Reeve, 2020). However, the question remains as to whether these guidelines are available to patients and such concepts highlighted in the practice or clinic.

It is important to understand the clinical inertia attached to deprescribing. This is defined as failing to act on inappropriate prescribing despite awareness of it due to stopping potentially inappropriate medicines (PIMs) being perceived as a problematic area for a number of reasons, including not wanting to conflict with other prescribers (especially specialists in their field), increased workloads and fear of unknown consequences (Anderson et al., 2014). It is important that you as a prescriber are aware of these barriers, but also work to overcome them so that deprescribing can be incorporated into good prescribing practices.

To conclude this section, we want to provide practical steps that can aid deprescribing within your practice. Scott et al. (2015) developed a five-step deprescribing algorithm to aid actioning deprescribing in practice. This comprises:

- determine all medicines the patient is currently taking and their indications;
- consider risk of medicine-induced harm in patients in determining the required intensity of deprescribing intervention;

- assess each medicine for its eligibility to be deprescribed;
- prioritise medicines to deprescribe;
- implement and monitor deprescribing regimen.

Medicine lists that highlight PIMs, such as STOPP-START and the Beers Criteria, can help prescribers identify potential medicines to deprescribe. The Beers Criteria is a list of PIMs that are usually best avoided in older patients; this may help providers identify medicines suitable for deprescribing (AGS, 2019). Prescribers can find further deprescribing support through websites such as deprescribing.org/ which hosts several deprescribing resources, algorithms and guidelines. Finally, deprescribing networks such as the English Deprescribing Network (EdeN) are great ways to connect with other prescribers and researchers who share a passion for improving prescribing through the use of deprescribing.

Summary

The chapter discussed your transition to nurse prescriber, the need for continuing professional development to support you and, finally, deprescribing. Within your transition from qualified nurse to nurse prescriber there are known challenges; this chapter aimed to provide you with some understanding of these and to suggest what steps could be taken to smooth the process. CPD can help support you in this transition to prescriber and, as in the final section of this chapter, support your deprescribing activities.

Deprescribing is defined as the process of stopping or reducing medicines with the aim of eliminating problematic (inappropriate) polypharmacy. Unfortunately, there are many potential barriers stopping any prescriber from initiating a deprescribing process – not only for you, as the healthcare professional, but also for the patient. These are discussed and explained. Practical steps that can aid deprescribing within your practice are outlined.

References

Ailabouni, N.J., Rebecca Weir, K., Reeve, E., Turner, J.T., Wilson Norton, J. and Gray, S.L. 2022. Barriers and enablers of older adults initiating a deprescribing conversation. *Patient Education and Counseling*. **105**, pp. 615–24.

American Geriatrics Society (AGS) 2019. Updated AGS Beers Criteria® for potentially inappropriate medication use in older adults. *Journal of the American Geriatrics Society*. **67**. pp. 674–94.

Anderson, K., Foster, M., Freeman, C., Luetsch, K. and Scott, I. 2017. Negotiating 'unmeasurable harm and benefit': Perspectives of general practitioners and consultant pharmacists on deprescribing in the primary care setting. *Qualitative Health Research*. **27**, pp. 1936–47.

Anderson, K., Stowasser, D., Freeman, C. and Scott, I. 2014. Prescriber barriers and enablers to minimising potentially inappropriate medications in adults: a systematic review and thematic synthesis. *BMJ Open*. **4**(12), e006544.

Benner, P. 1984. From novice to expert: Excellence and power in clinical nursing practice. *American Journal of Nursing.* **84**(12), p. 1480.

Bridges, W. 2004. *Transitions: Making Sense of Life's Changes.* Cambridge, MA: Da Capo Press.

Chief Medical Officer (CMO) 1998. A Review of Continuing Professional Development in General Practice: A Report by the Chief Medical Officer. London: DoH.

Doherty, A.J., Boland, P., Reed, J., Clegg, A.J., Stephani, A.M., Williams, N.H., Shaw, B., Hedgecoe, L., Hill, R. and Walker, L. 2020. Barriers and facilitators to deprescribing in primary care: A systematic review. *BJGP Open.* **4**(3).

Duchscher, J.E.B. 2008. A process of becoming: The stages of new nursing graduate professional role transition. *Journal of Continuing Education in Nursing.* **39**(10), pp. 441–50.

Duchscher, J.E.B. 2009. Transition shock: The initial stage of role adaptation for newly graduated registered nurses. *Journal of Advanced Nursing.* **65**(5), pp. 1103–13.

Duerden, M., Avery, T. and Payne, R. 2013. Polypharmacy and Medicines Optimisation: Making It Safe and Sound. London: King's Fund.

Field, S. 1998. Continuing professional development in primary care. *Medical Education.* **32**. pp. 564–6. Available at onlinelibrary.wiley.com/doi/full/10.1046/j.1365-2923.1998.00314.x (accessed 21 September 2023).

Fisher, J. 2008. Change happens to people. *Journal of Organisations and People.* **15**(4). pp. 4–8.

Henshaw, L. 2021. Transition to a health visitor role: A constructivist grounded theory. Dprof thesis. University of Derby.

Ibrahim, K., Cox, N.J., Stevenson, J.M., Lim, S., Fraser, S.D.S. and Roberts, H.C. 2021. A systematic review of the evidence for deprescribing interventions among older people living with frailty. *BMC Geriatrics.* **21**(1), art. 258.

Iyer, S., Naganathan, V., McLachlan, A.J. and Le Couteur, D.G. 2008. Medication withdrawal trials in people aged 65 years and older: A systematic review. *Drugs Aging.* **25**(12). pp. 1021–31.

Jansen, J., Naganathan, V., Carter, S.M., McLachlan, A.J., Nickel, B., Irwig, L., Bonner, C., Doust, J., Colvin, J., Heaney, A., Turner, R. and McCaffery, K. 2016. Too much medicine in older people? Deprescribing through shared decision making. *BMJ.* **353**, i2893.

Joseph, H.B., Issac, A., George, A.G., Gautam, G., Jiji, M. and Mondal, S. 2022. Transitional challenges and role of preceptor among new nursing graduates. *Journal of Caring Sciences.* **11**(2). pp. 56–63.

Kralik, D., Visentin, K. and Van Loon, A. 2006. Transition: A literature review. *Journal of Advanced Nursing.* **5**(3), pp. 320–9.

Kramer, M. 1974. *Reality Shock: Why Nurses Leave Nursing.* St Louis, MO: C.V. Mosby.

Kuntz, J.L., Kouch, L., Christian, D., Hu, W. and Peterson, P.L. 2019. Patient education and pharmacist consultation influence on nonbenzodiazepine sedative medication deprescribing success for older adults. *Permanente Journal.* **23**, pp. 18–161.

Linsky, A., Meterko, M., Bokhour, B.G., Stolzmann, K. and Simon, S.R. 2019. Deprescribing in the context of multiple providers: Understanding patient preferences. *American Journal of Managed Care.* **25**. pp. 192–8.

Martin, P., Tamblyn, R., Benedetti, A., Ahmed, S. and Tannenbaum, C. 2018. Effect of a pharmacist-led educational intervention on inappropriate medication prescriptions in older adults: The D-PRESCRIBE randomized clinical trial. *JAMA.* **320**(18). pp. 1889–98.

NMC 2018a. The Code: *Professional Standards of Practice and Behaviour for Nurses, Midwives and Nursing Associates.* Available at www.nmc.org.uk/globalassets/sitedocuments/nmc-publications/nmc-code.pdf (accessed 6 June 2023).

NMC 2018b. *Standards of Proficiency.* Available at www.nmc.org.uk/standards/standards-for-nurses/standards-of-proficiency-for-registered-nurses/ (accessed 6 June 2023).

Pirmohamed, M., James, S., Meakin, S., Green, C., Scott, A.K., Walley, T.J., Farrar, K., Park, B.K. and Breckenridge, A.M. 2004. Adverse drug reactions as a cause of admission to hospital: Prospective analysis of 18,820 patients. *BMJ.* **329**, pp. 15–19.

Reeve, E. 2020. Deprescribing tools: A review of the types of tools available to aid deprescribing in clinical practice. *Journal of Pharmacy Practice and Research.* **50**. pp. 98–107.

Reeve, E., To, J., Hendrix, I., Shakib, S., Roberts, M.S. and Wiese, M.D. 2013. Patient barriers to and enablers of deprescribing: A systematic review. *Drugs and Aging.* **30**(10). pp. 793–807.

RPS 2021. *A Competency Framework for All Prescribers.* Available at www.rpharms.com/resources/frameworks/prescribing-competency-framework/competency-framework (accessed 12 May 2023).

Scott, I.A., Hilmer, S.N., Reeve, E., Potter, K., Le Couteur, D., Rigby, D., Gnjidic, D., Del Mar, C.B., Roughead, E.E., Page, A., Jansen, J. and Martin, J.H. 2015. Reducing inappropriate polypharmacy: The process of deprescribing. *JAMA Internal Medicine.* **175**(5). pp. 827–34.

Wallis, K.A., Andrews, A. and Henderson, M. 2017. Swimming against the tide: Primary care physicians' views on deprescribing in everyday practice. *Annals of Family Medicine.* **15**. pp. 341–6.

Wenger, E. 1998. *Communities of Practice: Learning Meaning and Identity.* 6th ed. Cambridge: Cambridge University Press.

Wenger, E. 2010. Communities of practice and social learning systems: The career of a concept. In Blackmore, C. (Ed.), *Social Learning Systems and Communities of Practice.* London: Springer.

Woodward, M.C. 2003. Deprescribing: Achieving better health outcomes for older people through reducing medications. *Journal of Pharmacy Practice and Research.* **33**. pp. 323–8.

Wray, J., Watson, R., Gibson, H. and Barrett, D. 2021. Approaches used to enhance transition and retention for newly qualified nurses (NQNs): A rapid evidence assessment. *Nurse Education Today.* **98**. art. 104651.

Van Gennep, A. 1960. *The Rites of Passage.* London: Routledge and Kegan Paul.

Glossary of Terms

Administer: to give a medicine either by introduction into the body, whether by direct contact with the body or not (e.g., orally or by injection), or by external application (e.g., application of an impregnated dressing).

Adverse drug reaction: a response to a drug which is noxious and unintended, and which occurs at doses normally used in patients for prophylaxis, diagnosis, or therapy of disease or for the modification of physiologic function.

Antibiotics: specifically refer to those substances that target bacteria.

Antimicrobial: an umbrella term that encompasses chemical substances, of natural or synthetic origin, that suppress the growth of, or destroy, micro-organisms.

Antimicrobial resistance: when bacteria, viruses, fungi and parasites change over time and no longer respond to medicines.

Antimicrobial stewardship: an organisational or healthcare system-wide approach to promoting and monitoring judicious use of antimicrobials to preserve their future effectiveness.

Bioavailability: the proportion of any given drug that reaches the systemic circulation.

British National Formulary: contains a wide spectrum of information and advice on prescribing and pharmacology, along with specific facts and details about many available medicines.

British National Formulary for Children: published yearly and details the doses and uses of medicines in children from neonates to adolescents.

Calculating doses in paediatrics: body weight, body surface area, age.

Clinical commissioning groups (CCGs): see Integrated care boards.

Clinical management plan: a written or electronic therapeutic plan relating to a named patient which is integral to supplementary prescribing.

Cockcroft and Gault equation: measures creatinine clearance and therefore kidney function.

Communication skills: commonly adjunct to competence in physical assessment and examination.

Competency Framework for All Prescribers: a single competency framework; all prescribers need to maintain the same competencies in prescribing.

Concordant consultation: shared decision-making between you and the patient or their carer is essential for the relationship to be concordant.

Consultation: an opportunity for a patient and health professional to undertake a meeting reliant on discussion and collaboration.

Consultation models: commonly used to absorb structure to a clinical consultation to help refrain the consultation from deteriorating into what can be perceived as disarray and subsequent dysfunction, potentially leading to an ineffectual outcome.

Continuing education: a largely passive activity, such as attendance at conferences and courses.

Continuing professional development (CPD): an active process which involves not just attending a training event, but also reflection as to how this might change your practice.

Controlled drugs: drugs that are subject to high levels of regulation as a result of government decisions about those drugs that can be especially addictive and harmful.

Crown reports: a number of reports and reviews that led to the formal introduction of prescribing by healthcare professionals in addition to doctors and dentists.

Cumberlege report: this 1986 report discusses all aspects of nursing in the community, making recommendations on each aspect.

Deprescribing: a systematic process of identifying and discontinuing drugs where harms outweigh benefits within the context of an individual patient's care goals and their current level of functioning.

Differential diagnosis: where you, as the prescriber and healthcare professional, weigh up the likelihood of one condition over another.

Drug interactions: a reaction between two (or more) drugs or between a drug and a food, beverage, or supplement.

Drug tariff: this provides information on what will be paid to contractors for NHS Services, including the cost of drugs and appliances supplied against an NHS prescription, but also remuneration to NHS contractors such as pharmacies.

Duty of care: providing information about the potential for risk of harm and also ensuring patients have information about the likely benefit of the treatments prescribed to them in order to promote informed consent.

Electronic Medicines Compendium (EMC): the most up-to-date, approved and regulated information source on medicines and patient information for licensed drugs.

Epidemiology collaboration (CKD-EPI): a method of calculating drug doses in patients with renal impairment.

Excipient: an inactive substance that serves as the vehicle or medium for a drug or other active substance. They are things like colouring agents, preservatives and fillers.

Formularies: in the UK, formularies exist to specify which drugs are available on the NHS for particular groups of prescribers.

Framework: a system that guides and supports you use when you are dealing with an activity such as prescribing.

Generic prescribing: uses what is called the international non-proprietary name (INN).

Half-life: the time taken to reduce the plasma concentration to half of its original value.

Independent prescribing: prescribing by an appropriate practitioner (e.g., doctor, dentist, nurse, pharmacist etc.) responsible and accountable for the assessment of patients with undiagnosed or diagnosed conditions and for decisions about the clinical management required, including prescribing.

Integrated care boards (ICBs): replaced clinical commissioning groups (CCGs) in the NHS in England from 1 July 2022. They may make recommendations or even offer incentives to prescribe in a certain way and to increase the amount of generic prescribing.

Learn from patient safety events (Lfpse): an NHS service for the recording and analysis of patient safety events that occur in healthcare.

Medicines adherence: describes the extent to which a patient's medicines use matches the agreed recommendations from the prescriber.

Medicines optimisation: a person-centred approach to safe and effective medicines use.

Multidisciplinary teams (MDTs): many healthcare professions such as medics, nurses, pharmacists and physiotherapists in one building, working together for the benefit of the patient.

National Patient Safety Agency (NPSA): this agency collected information on medication errors using the National Reporting and Learning System (NRLS, see below). Through this, they identified the medicines most frequently associated with severe harm.

National Reporting and Learning System (NRLS): collected information on safety incidents to enable analysis and generate learning to improve the state of care. Taken over by Lfpse.

Nurse Prescribers' Formulary: initially a list of products that were permitted to be prescribed by community nurses who had undergone the necessary training to enable the nurse to prescribe in areas such as minor injuries, minor ailments, health promotion and palliative care.

Off-label prescribing: prescribing a licensed medicine for use in an unlicensed condition or outside the terms of its licence in some other way – such as prescribing a medicine licensed for adults but for a child.

Patient decision aid: an evidence-based resource designed to help and support patients to make decisions when there are choices about different treatments.

Patient group direction (PGD): provides a legal framework that allows some registered health professionals to supply and/or administer specified medicines to a pre-defined group of patients.

Patient information leaflet (PIL): This is the package insert the patient receives with their prescribed medicines. See also electronic medicines compendium.

Patient-specific direction (PSD): an instruction to administer a medicine to a list of specifically named patients where each patient on the list has been individually assessed by a prescriber.

Pharmacodynamics: the effect of the drug on the body.

Pharmacokinetics: the effect of the body on the drug.

PGD: see Patient group direction.

Prescribe: in the strict legal sense, as used in the Medicines Act of 1968: (i) to order in writing the supply of a prescription-only medicine for a named patient; (ii) to authorise by means of an NHS prescription the supply of any medicine (not just a prescription-only medicine) at public expense.

Prescribing analysis and cost (PACT): available since the end of the 1980s, it analyses every prescription that is dispensed.

Primary care networks (PCNs): where groups of practices work together; may also have an influence on the overall choice of medicines for particular conditions.

PSD: see Patient-specific directions.

Quality and outcomes frameworks (QOF): intended to improve the quality of care patients are given by rewarding practices for the quality of their provision to their patients, based on several indicators across a range of key areas of clinical care and public health.

Red flags: alarm symptoms and issues, including prescribing for patients with complex care needs or where high-risk treatments are likely to be prescribed and consultation where it is uncertain if the person has capacity.

Remote prescribing: occurs in the context of the prescriber and the patient being physically or geographically remote from each other.

Risk of harm: associated with medicine-taking; typically refers to the likelihood of experiencing a side-effect associated with a treatment.

Royal Pharmaceutical Society (RPS): Publisher of the competency framework for all prescibers.

Safeguarding: defined in the Care Act (2014) as protecting an adult's right to live in safety, free from abuse and neglect.

Side-effect: an undesired effect that occurs when the medication is administered, regardless of the dose.

START: a screening tool designed to alert a practitioner to the right treatment.

STOPP: a screening tool intended for treatment of older persons, including covering potentially inappropriate prescriptions.

Supplementary prescribing: a voluntary partnership between an independent prescriber (a doctor or dentist) and a supplementary prescriber to implement an agreed patient-specific clinical management plan (CMP) with the patient's agreement.

Supply: to provide a medicine directly to a patient or carer for administration.

Teratogen: any agent that causes an abnormality following foetal exposure during pregnancy.

Therapeutic index: the ratio of the dose that produces toxicity to the dose that produces a clinically desired or effective response.

Transition to prescribing role: transition from one healthcare professional role to another which highlights issues with identity and autonomy as additional important concepts.

TYPE A ADRs: augmented, related to the pharmacological properties of the drug.

TYPE B ADRs: bizarre or unexpected and unpredictable.

TYPE C ADRs: chronic, develops after chronic use.

TYPE D ADRs: delayed, occurs long after use.

TYPE E ADRs: end of use, effects after stopping the medicine.

Unlicensed medicine: means simply that a licence for this medicine has not been granted but it may still be appropriate to prescribe it.

Appendix 1

 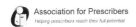 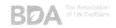 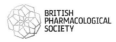

 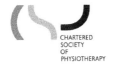 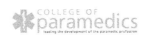 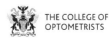

 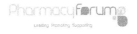 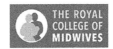 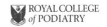

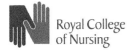

The competency framework for all prescribers

This competency framework for all prescribers sets out what good prescribing looks like. Its implementation and maintenance are important in informing and improving practice, development, standard of care and safety (for both the prescriber and patient).

Prescribers are encouraged to use their own professional codes of conduct, standards and guidance alongside this framework. Prescribers are also responsible for practising within their own scope of practice and competence, including delegating where appropriate, seeking support when required and using their acquired knowledge, skills and professional judgement.

It is important to recognise that healthcare professionals need to apply professionalism to all aspects of their practice. The principles of professionalism are the same across the professions and these are behaviours that healthcare professionals should always be demonstrating, not just for prescribing. There are elements of wider professional practice that will impact on how healthcare professionals behave when they prescribe. These include the importance of maintaining a patient-centred approach when speaking to patients/carers, maintaining confidentiality, communication skills, leadership, the need for reflection, maintaining competency and continuing professional development, and the importance of forming networks for support and learning.

Structure of the framework

Domains

The competencies within the framework are presented as two domains and describe the knowledge, skill, behaviour, activity, or outcome that prescribers should demonstrate:

Domain one – the consultation

This domain looks at the competencies that the prescriber should demonstrate during the consultation.

Domain two – prescribing governance

This domain focuses on the competencies that the prescriber should demonstrate with respect to prescribing governance.

Competency and supporting statements

Within the two domains there are ten competencies, as shown in Figure A.1.

Each of these competencies contains several supporting statements related to the prescriber role which describe the activity or outcome that the prescriber should actively and routinely demonstrate.

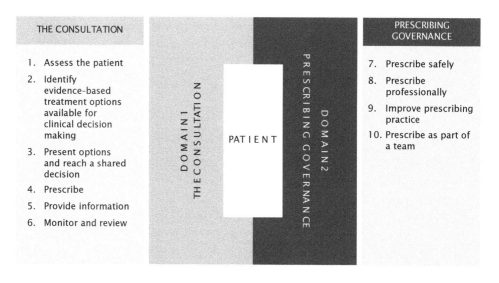

THE CONSULTATION

1. Assess the patient
2. Identify evidence-based treatment options available for clinical decision making
3. Present options and reach a shared decision
4. Prescribe
5. Provide information
6. Monitor and review

PRESCRIBING GOVERNANCE

7. Prescribe safely
8. Prescribe professionally
9. Improve prescribing practice
10. Prescribe as part of a team

DOMAIN 1 THE CONSULTATION

PATIENT

DOMAIN 2 PRESCRIBING GOVERNANCE

Figure A.1 The Competency Framework for all Prescribers

Please note

- The framework competencies and supporting statements are not in any particular order. The numbering is mainly to support mapping purposes and does not reflect the level of importance of the statement. They are not designed to be used as a script or in isolation as they may overlap with others.
- Due to the generic nature of the framework, it may be that not every competency or supporting statement is relevant to your practice or setting. However, you should still be able to consider how you could demonstrate the supporting statement.

Further information

The further information sections under each competency provide prescribers with information and examples (list not exhaustive or definitive), which provide clarity and meaning to the supporting statements. The recommendation for this framework is to use it alongside any relevant further information sections to support implementation into practice.

For further supporting resources, please see the RPS website here: https://www.rpharms.com/cfap

Domain one: The consultation

1. Assess the patient

Statements supporting the competency

1.1. Undertakes the consultation in an appropriate setting[a].

1.2. Considers patient dignity, capacity, consent and confidentiality[b].

1.3. Introduces self and prescribing role to the patient/carer and confirms patient/carer identity.

1.4. Assesses the communication needs of the patient/carer and adapts[c] consultation appropriately.

1.5. Demonstrates good consultation skills[d] and builds rapport with the patient/carer.

1.6. Takes and documents an appropriate medical, psychosocial and medication history[e] including allergies and intolerances.

1.7. Undertakes and documents an appropriate clinical assessment[f].

1.8. Identifies and addresses potential vulnerabilities[g] that may be causing the patient/carer to seek treatment.

1.9. Accesses and interprets all available and relevant patient records to ensure knowledge of the patient's management to date.

1.10. Requests and interprets relevant investigations necessary to inform treatment options.

1.11. Makes, confirms or understands, and documents the working or final diagnosis by systematically considering the various possibilities (differential diagnosis).

1.12. Understands the condition(s) being treated, their natural progression, and how to assess their severity, deterioration and anticipated response to treatment.

1.13. Reviews adherence (and non-adherence[h]) to, and effectiveness of, current medicines.

1.14. Refers to or seeks guidance from another member of the team, a specialist or appropriate information source when necessary.

Further information on the supporting statements for competency 1

[a]Appropriate setting includes location, environment and medium.

[b]In line with legislation, best practice, regulatory standards and contractual requirements.

[c]Adapts for language, age, capacity, learning disability and physical or sensory impairments.

[d]Good consultation skills include actively listening, using positive body language, asking open questions, remaining non-judgemental, and exploring the patient's/carer's ideas, concerns and expectations.

[e]Medication history includes current and previously prescribed (and non-prescribed) medicines, vaccines, on-line medicines, over-the-counter medicines, vitamins, dietary supplements, herbal products, complementary remedies, recreational/illicit drugs, alcohol and tobacco.

[f]Clinical assessment includes observations, psychosocial assessments and physical examinations.

[g]Safeguarding children and vulnerable adults (possible signs of abuse, neglect, or exploitation), and focusing on both the patient's physical and mental health, particularly if vulnerabilities may lead them to seek treatment unnecessarily or for the wrong reasons.

[h]Non-adherence may be intentional or non-intentional.

2. Identify evidence-based treatment options available for clinical decision making

Statements supporting the competency

2.1. Considers both non-pharmacological[a] and pharmacological treatment approaches.

2.2. Considers all pharmacological treatment options including optimising doses as well as stopping treatment (appropriate polypharmacy and deprescribing).

2.3. Assesses the risks and benefits to the patient of taking or not taking a medicine or treatment.

2.4. Applies understanding of the pharmacokinetics and pharmacodynamics of medicines, and how these may be altered by individual patient factors[b].

2.5. Assesses how co-morbidities, existing medicines, allergies, intolerances, contraindications and quality of life impact on management options.

2.6. Considers any relevant patient factors[c] and their potential impact on the choice and formulation of medicines, and the route of administration.

2.7. Accesses, critically evaluates, and uses reliable and validated sources of information.

2.8. Stays up to date in own area of practice and applies the principles of evidence-based practice[d].

2.9. Considers the wider perspective including the public health issues related to medicines and their use, and promoting health.

2.10. Understands antimicrobial resistance and the roles of infection prevention, control and antimicrobial stewardship measures.

Further information on the supporting statements for competency 2

[a]Non-pharmacological treatment approaches include no treatment, social prescribing and wellbeing/lifestyle changes.

[b]Individual patient factors include genetics, age, renal impairment and pregnancy.

[c]Relevant patient factors include ability to swallow, disability, visual impairment, frailty, dexterity, religion, beliefs and intolerances.

[d]Evidence-based practice includes clinical and cost-effectiveness.

3. Present options and reach a shared decision

Statements supporting the competency

3.1. Actively involves and works with the patient/carer to make informed choices and agree a plan that respects the patient's/carer's preferences[a].

3.2. Considers and respects patient diversity, background, personal values and beliefs about their health, treatment and medicines, supporting the values of equality and inclusivity, and developing cultural competence.[b]

3.3. Explains the material risks and benefits, and rationale behind management options in a way the patient/carer understands, so that they can make an informed choice.

3.4. Assesses adherence in a non-judgemental way; understands the reasons for non-adherence[c] and how best to support the patient/carer.

3.5. Builds a relationship which encourages appropriate prescribing and not the expectation that a prescription will be supplied.

3.6. Explores the patient's/carer's understanding of a consultation and aims for a satisfactory outcome for the patient/carer and prescriber.

Further in formation on the supporting statements for competency 3

[a]Preferences include patient's/carer's right to decline or limit treatment.

[b]In line with legislation requirements which apply to equality, diversity and inclusion.

[c]Non-adherence may be intentional or non-intentional.

4. Prescribe

Statements supporting the competency

4.1. Prescribes a medicine or device[a] with up-to-date awareness of its actions, indications, dose, contraindications, interactions, cautions and adverse effects.

4.2. Understands the potential for adverse effects and takes steps to recognise, and manage them, whilst minimising risk.

4.3. Understands and uses relevant national, regional and local frameworks[b] for the use of medicines.

4.4. Prescribes generic medicines where practical and safe for the patient, and knows when medicines should be prescribed by branded product.

4.5. Accurately completes and routinely checks calculations relevant to prescribing and practical dosing.

4.6. Prescribes appropriate quantities and at appropriate intervals necessary[c] to reduce the risk of unnecessary waste.

4.7. Recognises potential misuse of medicines; minimises risk[d] and manages using appropriate processes.

4.8. Uses up-to-date information about the availability, pack sizes, storage conditions, excipients and costs of prescribed medicines.

4.9. Electronically generates and/or writes legible, unambiguous and complete prescriptions which meet legal requirements.

4.10. Effectively uses the systems[e] necessary to prescribe medicines.

4.11. Prescribes unlicensed and off-label medicines where legally permitted, and unlicensed medicines only if satisfied that an alternative licensed medicine would not meet the patient's clinical needs.

4.12. Follows appropriate safeguards if prescribing medicines that are unlicensed, off-label, or outside standard practice.

4.13. Documents accurate, legible and contemporaneous clinical records[f].

4.14. Effectively and securely communicates information[g] to other healthcare professionals involved in the patient's care, when sharing or transferring care and prescribing responsibilities, within and across all care settings.

Further information on the supporting statements for competency 4

[a]'Medicine' or 'device' includes all products (including necessary co-prescribing of infusion sets, devices, diluents and mediums) that can be prescribed, supplied or recommended for purchase.

[b]Frameworks include local formularies, care pathways, protocols and professional guidelines, as well as evidence-based guidelines from relevant national, regional and local committees.

[c]Amount necessary for a complete course, until next review or prescription supply.

[d]Minimises risk by ensuring appropriate safeguards are in place.

[e]Systems include medicine charts, decision support tools and electronic prescribing systems. Also, awareness and avoidance of potential system errors.

[f]Records include prescribing decisions, history, diagnosis, clinical indications, discussions, advice given, examinations, findings, interventions, action plans, safety-netting, referrals, monitoring and follow ups.

[g]Information about clinical conditions, medicines and their current use (where necessary and with valid consent). Ensuring that private and personal data is protected and communicated securely in line with relevant legislation/regulations.

5. Provide information

Statements supporting the competency

5.1. Assesses health literacy of the patient/carer and adapts appropriately to provide clear, understandable and accessible information[a].

5.2. Checks the patient's/carer's understanding of the discussions had, actions needed and their commitment to the management plan[b].

5.3. Guides the patient/carer on how to identify reliable sources[c] of information about their condition, medicines and treatment.

5.4. Ensures the patient/carer knows what to do if there are any concerns about the management of their condition, if the condition deteriorates or if there is no improvement in a specific timeframe.[d]

5.5. Encourages and supports the patient/carer to take responsibility for their medicines and self-manage their condition.

Further information on the supporting statements for Competency 5

[a]Information about their management, treatment, medicines (what they are for, how to use them, safe storage, disposal, expected duration of treatment, possible unwanted effects and what to do if they arise) monitoring and follow-up—in written and/or verbal form.

[b]Management plan includes treatment, medicines, monitoring and follow-up.

[c]Reliable sources include the medicine's patient information leaflet.

[d]Includes safety-netting advice on when and how to seek help through appropriate signposting and referral.

6. Monitor and review

Statements supporting the competency

6.1. Establishes and maintains a plan for reviewing[a] the patient's treatment.

6.2. Establishes and maintains a plan to monitor[b] the effectiveness of treatment and potential unwanted effects.

6.3. Adapts the management plan in response to on-going monitoring and review of the patient's condition and preferences.

6.4. Recognises and reports suspected adverse events to medicines and medical devices using appropriate reporting systems[c].

Further information on the supporting statements for competency 6

[a]Plan for reviewing includes safety-netting appropriate follow-up or referral.

[b]Plan for monitoring includes safety-netting monitoring requirements and responsibilities, for example, by the prescriber, patient/carer or other healthcare professional.

[c]Reporting systems include following established clinical governance procedures and the Medicines and Healthcare products Regulatory Agency (MHRA) Yellow Card scheme.

Domain two: Prescribing governance

7. Prescribe safely

Statements supporting the competency

7.1. Prescribes within own scope of practice, and recognises the limits of own knowledge and skill.

7.2. Knows about common types and causes of medication and prescribing errors, and knows how to minimise their risk.

7.3. Identifies and minimises potential risks associated with prescribing via remote methods[a].

7.4. Recognises when safe prescribing processes are not in place and acts to minimise risks[b].

7.5. Keeps up to date with emerging safety concerns related to prescribing.

7.6. Reports near misses and critical incidents, as well as medication and prescribing errors using appropriate reporting systems, whilst regularly reviewing practice[c] to prevent recurrence.

Further information on the supporting statements for competency 7

[a]Remote methods include telephone, email, video or communication via a third party.

[b]Minimising risks include using or developing governance processes that support safe prescribing, particularly in areas of high risk such as transfer of information about medicines and prescribing of repeat medicines.

[c]Reviewing practice include clinical audits.

8. Prescribe Professionally

Statements supporting the competency

8.1. Ensures confidence and competence to prescribe are maintained.

8.2. Accepts personal responsibility and accountability for prescribing[a] and clinical decisions, and understands the legal and ethical implications.

8.3. Knows and works within legal and regulatory frameworks[b] affecting prescribing practice.

8.4. Makes prescribing decisions based on the needs of patients and not the prescriber's personal views.

8.5. Recognises and responds to factors[c] that might influence prescribing.

8.6. Works within the NHS, organisational, regulatory and other codes of conduct when interacting with the pharmaceutical industry.

Further information on the supporting statements for competency 8

[a]Prescribing decisions include when prescribing under a shared care protocol/agreement.

[b]Frameworks for prescribing controlled drugs, unlicensed and off-label medicines, supplementary prescribing, and prescribing for self, close family and friends.

[c]Factors include interactions with pharmaceutical industry, media, patients/carers, colleagues, cognitive bias, financial gain, prescribing incentive schemes, switches and targets.

9. Improve Prescribing Practice

Statements supporting the competency

9.1. Improves by reflecting on own and others' prescribing practice, and by acting upon feedback and discussion.

9.2. Acts upon inappropriate or unsafe prescribing practice using appropriate processes[a].

9.3. Understands and uses available tools[b] to improve prescribing practice.

9.4. Takes responsibility for own learning and continuing professional development relevant to the prescribing role.[c]

9.5. Makes use of networks for support and learning.

9.6. Encourages and supports others with their prescribing practice and continuing professional development.[d]

9.7. Considers the impact of prescribing on sustainability, as well as methods of reducing the carbon footprint and environmental impact of any medicine.[e]

Further information on the supporting statements for competency 9

[a]Processes include whistleblowing, regulatory and professional guidance, and employer procedures.

[b]Tools include supervision, observation of practice and clinical assessment skills, portfolios, workplace competency-based assessments, questionnaires, prescribing data analysis, audits, case-based discussions, personal formularies and actively seeking regular patient and peer feedback.

[c]By continuously reviewing, reflecting, identifying gaps, planning, acting, applying and evidencing learning or competencies.

[d]By considering mentoring, leadership and workforce development (for example, becoming a Designated Prescribing Practitioner).

[e]Methods of reducing a medicine's carbon footprint and environmental impact include proper disposal of medicine/device/equipment waste, recycling schemes, avoiding overprescribing and waste through regular reviews, deprescribing, dose and device optimisation.

10. Prescribe as part of A team

Statements supporting the competency

10.1. Works collaboratively[a] as part of a multidisciplinary team to ensure that the transfer and continuity of care (within and across all care settings) is developed and not compromised.

10.2. Establishes relationships with other professionals based on understanding, trust and respect for each other's roles in relation to the patient's care.

10.3. Agrees the appropriate level of support and supervision for their role as a prescriber.

10.4. Provides support and advice[b] to other prescribers or those involved in administration of medicines where appropriate.

Further in formation on the supporting statements for competency 10

[a]Working collaboratively may also include keeping the patient/carer informed or prescribing under a shared care protocol/agreement.

[b]Advice may include any specific instructions for administration, advice to be given to the patient/carer and monitoring required immediately after administration.

Appendix 2
Antibiotic 'superbugs'

This appendix describes three common 'superbugs' that you, as a prescriber, should know how to manage and sets out some factors relating to prescribing that help minimise the impact of these superbugs and reinforce the need for prescribers to prioritise antimicrobial stewardship.

Clostridium difficile

Around 2–25 per cent of patients taking antibiotics will experience diarrhoea associated with antibiotic usage; this is a common side-effect (Bartlett, 2002). About a fifth of these cases of antibiotic-related diarrhoea are caused because the antibiotics bring about a disruption of the bowel microbiota and mucosal integrity, which in turn results in an overgrowth of a bacteria called clostridium difficile (Steele et al., 2015; NICE, 2022). Clostridium difficile is a gram-positive bacteria; the diarrhoea it causes is not from the colonisation of the bacteria itself, but from the build-up of toxins it produces damaging the lining of the colon.

Due to the association with antibiotic use (antibiotic exposure almost always precedes infection) you, as a nurse prescriber, must employ the principles of antimicrobial stewardship discussed in chapter 6 when prescribing antibiotics and managing this condition (HSA, 2022a).

Some key principles to consider include:

- infection prevention and control;
- hands must be washed using soap and water because alcohol gel is not effective against the spores that cause this infection;
- in-patients with clostridium difficile should be nursed in source isolation;
- PPE requirements include the use of gloves and aprons.

Pharmaceutical treatment and review

When caring for patients with a clostridium difficile infection you should undertake a medicine review, paying particular attention to the requirements for antibiotics that are not essential for a non-clostridium difficile infection indication, laxatives, PPIs, diuretics, ACE-inhibitors and NSAIDs (HSA, 2022a).

First-line treatment for a clostridium difficile infection is vancomycin 125mg orally four times a day for ten days. If this is not effective then Fidaxomicin, 200mg orally twice a day for ten days can be prescribed as a second-line treatment. You, as the prescriber, must use your clinical judgement to review the effectiveness of initial treatment and if these treatments are not effective, it is recommended that you seek expert advice on more suitable antibiotic regimes (NICE, 2022).

Methicillin-Resistant Staphylococcus Aureus (MRSA)

This has a long history of notoriety and was a 'media star' in the early 2000s with promises from politicians, such as Tony Blair, that they would eliminate the bug from hospitals. The prevention of transmission of MRSA in healthcare settings remains an important concern for you and other nurse prescribers. Staphylococcus aureus is a common gram-positive bacterium that can colonise parts of the body, such as the skin, gut or nose, without symptoms being present.

Since the 1960s, strains of Staphylococcus aureus have been identified that are resistant to several commonly used antibacterial agents including beta-lactam antibacterials and flucloxacillin (Prestinaci et al., 2015). These bacteria can be responsible for common hospital-acquired infections such as surgical site infections, bloodstream infections, sepsis and pneumonias. There has also been an increase of these infections in the community (community-acquired MRSA or CA-MRSA).

In the first instance you need to know and understand the strategies to minimise the transmission and poor health outcomes associated with MRSA. These include the application of standard infection prevention policies, such as handwashing, use of PPE and contact precautions. Source isolation for those infected may also be a requirement. Cleaning and decontamination of clinical areas is essential to manage the risk of transmission.

Screening for MRSA colonisation may be advised in some populations, such as patients scheduled for surgery, but it is not a requirement to routinely screen staff for MRSA colonisation.

When colonisation has been identified, treatments for decolonisation might include the following:

- mupirocin for nasal decolonisation;
- chlorhexidine for body decolonisation;
- alternatives (e.g., octenidine) where mupirocin and chlorhexidine are not feasible can be considered – for example, due to resistance;
- oral doxycycline, trimethoprim, ciprofloxacin, or co-trimoxazole can be considered for lower urinary-tract infections caused by MRSA according to susceptibility (BNF 2022).

Carbapenemase-Producing Enterobacterales

Carbapenemase-producing Enterobacterales (CPE) are a significant threat to healthcare and most healthcare trusts in England have identified patients colonised with CPE in recent years (HSA, 2022b). CPE are gram-positive bacteria that have become resistant to carbapenems and pose a significant threat to public health and treatment pathways (HSA, 2022b). There are limited treatments for those infected and treatment options need review by infection specialists. Procedures such as decolonisation are not recommended due to the increase in risk of antimicrobial resistance. Key risk management strategies include the following:

- screening;
- monitoring and surveillance;
- managing transmission;
- cleaning and decontamination;
- antimicrobial stewardship.

As a nurse prescriber, you need to be aware of the increased risk to patients exposed to broad-spectrum antibiotic courses that may increase the risk of CPE. These include cephalosporins, glycopeptides and piperacillin or tazobactam. The use of carbapenems within the past month is also a noteworthy risk factor. Consequently, it is essential for nurse prescribers to embed antimicrobial stewardship into typical practice to minimise inappropriate use of broad-spectrum antibiotics, including carbapenems. This is one of the most essential mitigation strategies against this drug-resistant bacteria that we currently have.

References

Bartlett, J.G. 2002. Clinical practice: Antibiotic-associated diarrhoea. *New England Journal of Medicine.* **346**(5). pp. 334–9.

BNF 2022. *British National Formulary: Treatment Summaries – MRSA.* Available at bnf.nice.org.uk/treatment-summaries/mrsa/ and www.nhs.uk/conditions/mrsa/ (accessed 31 January 2023).

Health Security Agency (HSA) 2022a. *Clostridioides difficile infection: Updated guidance on management and treatment.* Available at assets.publishing.service.gov.uk/government/uploads/system/uploads/attachment_data/file/1118277/UKHSA-CDI-guideline-july-2022_DRAFT.pdf (accessed 21 September 2023).

Health Security Agency 2022b. *Framework of Actions to Contain Carbapenemase-producing Enterobacterales.* Available at assets.publishing.service.gov.uk/government/uploads/system/uploads/attachment_data/file/1107705/Framework_of_actions_to_contain_CPE.pdf (accessed 31 May 2023). Guidelines to be updated.

NICE 2022. *Clinical Knowledge Summary: Diarrhoea – Antibiotic Associated.* Available at cks.nice.org.uk/topics/diarrhoea-antibiotic-associated/background-information/definition/ (accessed 6 November 2022).

Prestinaci, F., Pezzotti, P. and Pantosti, A. 2015. Antimicrobial resistance: A global multifaceted phenomenon. *Pathogens and Global Health*. **109**(7), pp. 309–18. Available at www.ncbi.nlm.nih.gov/pmc/articles/PMC4768623/#__ffn_sectitle (accessed 31 May 2023).

Steele, S.R., McCormick, J., Melton, G.B. Paquette, I., Rivadeneira, D.E., Stewart, D., Donald Buie, W. and Rafferty, J. 2015. Practice parameters for the management of Clostridium difficile infection. *Diseases of the Colon and Rectum*. **58**(1), pp. 10–24.

Appendix 3
Calculations

Barry Strickland-Hodge

Introduction

There are a number of very good books devoted to supporting nurses and others in choosing the appropriate doses for administration of drugs. Often this is choosing the correct volume from ampoules. There are also a number of examples in Appendix 1 of our sister book entitled *Practical Prescribing for Medical Students* (Bradbury and Strickland-Hodge, 2014). However, there are very few that discuss this with the prescriber in mind.

The *Competency Framework for All Prescribers* (RPS, 2021) mentions calculations. In Competency 4, Prescribe, supporting statement 4.5 says: 'Accurately completes and routinely checks calculations relevant to prescribing and practical dosing' and 4.6 states: 'Prescribes appropriate quantities and at appropriate intervals necessary to reduce the risk of unnecessary waste'.

You may consider maths is not your area of expertise, but we have to try to think in terms that put calculating doses into context. You may call it maths, but surely it just part of your prescribing role. If something seems to be too complicated then ask for support. To me there are three ways of approaching doses: common sense, which suggests the dose is too high or too low; the next step is back to first principles – I realise the words can sound complicated but it is the best way; finally, there are short cuts – although these will be mentioned, it is important that you use the first two options if you are not familiar with the doses of the medicine you are to prescribe. Many units are simply one to be taken three time a day or similar for a set period such as five days or a month; however, in the hospital or clinic setting you may need to calculate a dose for an injection where the content of the ampoule is not the dose you want. Again, this is generally for administration but if you are to ensure the correct amount is given by a third party on the ward then you will need to write the prescription explicitly.

In this short section, I will try to offer some guidance as to how to tackle calculations in various forms, some of which you may not come across in practice as a prescriber – but if you do you will know what to do. Remember, common sense and experience are important but first principles are essential.

We'll start at the very basic level so please skip this if it's too basic for you.

Mass

Box A.1 shows the various important divisions of mass and their appropriate abbreviations.

Box A.1

Mass

1000 grams in 1 kilogram
1000mg in 1 gram
1000 micrograms in 1mg
1000 nanograms in 1 microgram
Grams can be abbreviated to 'g'
Milligrams can be abbreviated to 'mg'
Micrograms should **always** be written in full (you may see mcg or µg but this is not appropriate in prescribing situations and can easily be misinterpreted).
Nanograms should **always** be written in full (you may see ng or ɳg but again this is not appropriate in prescribing and can be misinterpreted).
Decimal places must be avoided. 500mg should not be written as 0.5g, as of course this could be read as 5mg, especially if handwritten.

Volume

Box A.2 shows the same as in **Box A.1** but for volume.

Box A.2

Volume

1000mL in 1 litre
It is more common now to see litre as a capital L so
Millilitres can be abbreviated to mL
Litres can be abbreviated to L

Concentration

You may have come across ointments, liquid mixtures or powder mixtures that end with the letters ww, wv or vv (if not it might be an idea to have a look at some ointment tubes and eye drops). See **Box A.3** for examples.

W stands for weight and V stands for volume.

Box A.3

Something like eye drops may have the letters w/v after the active ingredient or each ingredient if more than one. This stands for weight in (or per) volume. So potentially a dry ingredient (w) has been added to a liquid (v) to create the solution.

An example could be a 5% solution w/v which means 5g in 100 (per cent) mL.

If there is more than one active ingredient you may see the letters after each one.

If two liquids have been added together to create a solution then there may be the letter v/v after the active ingredient. This stands for volume in or per volume.

For example, a 5% v/v solution = 5mL in 100mL

Atropine eye drops are 0.5% v/v

Which is 0.5mL of atropine liquid in 100mL of solution.

Finally, if two dry ingredients have been added together to create say an ointment then the letters w/w will stand for weight in or per weight.

Some simple examples are:

Betnovate RD cream says it is betamethasone valerate 0.025% w/w. It also says there are 0.25mg in a gram of the cream. Is this the same thing?
1 gram is 1000 milligrams.
So, 0.25mg in 1000mg of cream is 0.025mg in 100mg (ten times less) or 0.025% w/w

Calculation A.1

What dose of salbutamol syrup would be required for a 40kg child when the recommended dose is 100 micrograms per kilogram three times a day?

Answer A.1

Dose = 100 micrograms × 40kg = 4000 micrograms.

(Salbutamol syrup is available as a 2mg/5mL solution so it is more sensible to express this answer in milligrams, i.e., 4000 micrograms ÷ 1000 = 4mg)

The dose on the prescription is therefore TWO 5mL spoonsful three times a day.

Calculation A.2

An adult patient is prescribed 225mg of phenytoin liquid 90mg/5mL. What volume needs to be given if you have 90mg in 5mL?

Answer A.2

Using first principles:

You have 90mg in 5mL

Which is 1mg in (5 ÷ 90) mL = 0.05555mL

So,

225mg will be in 225 × 0.05555mL = 12.5mL

Another way is to say;

what we want (225mg) divided by what we have (90mg) multiplied by the volume (5mL)

This gives is 225/90 × 5 which is 12.5mL

Some further simple calculations

Calculation A.3 and A4 (answers following the calculations as answer A3 and A4)

One of your 60-year-old male patients whom you have managed for some time in the practice has asked you to telephone him at home as he has a recurrent chest infection which affects his chronic obstructive pulmonary disease. You check his notes and from your experience of his condition decide to prescribe the antibiotics and oral steroids he has had before:

Amoxicillin 500mg capsules – one capsule three times a day (eight-hourly) for seven days and remind him to complete the whole course. He usually takes one first thing in the morning one in the middle of the day and one last thing at night. Not exactly every eight hours but this is the easiest to manage.

Prednisolone 5mg tablets – six tablets daily in the morning for seven days (which will need no reducing doses as it is only for seven days).

1. What is the daily dose of amoxicillin in g?
2. How many capsules of amoxicillin should be supplied in total for the week?
3. What is the total daily dose of prednisolone in mg?
4. How many tablets of prednisolone need to be supplied for seven days?

Calculation A.4

A 50-year-old Caucasian male patient was diagnosed with hypertension some time ago. Prior to a review, and as requested, the patient has been recording his blood pressure at home three times a day (using a standardised blood pressure monitor) for three days. The patient sends you the monitoring results via email in an Excel sheet and they show his blood pressure is not as controlled as either of you would like.

Following the relevant guidelines, you would like to prescribe an ACE inhibitor. You will need to discuss the treatment, the risk and benefits of keeping his blood pressure within normal parameters, any potential side-effects and how to manage them or who to contact if this becomes unmanageable. You have already built up a good rapport with the patient and are sure he will adhere but it is important that the consultation is concordant and that the patient listens and is part of the decision-making process. This is a telephone conversation so it is more difficult to observe any facial expressions.

He has no renal impairment or other contraindications to treatment.

You discuss with him a prescription for an ACE inhibitor as he is in the right age group (under 55) and racial group Caucasian. You both agree to a two-week trial of ramipril 2.5mg tablets once daily with a review at that point. If any side-effects are manageable you will consider the next step with the patient. You check the BNF which has a section not only on ramipril, but also on angiotensin-converting enzyme inhibitors (ACE inhibitors) which you consult.

a.   How many ramipril 2.5mg tablets will you prescribe for two weeks?
b.   How many mg of ramipril will the patient have taken over one week?

You review the patient after the two weeks and talk, first, about how easy it was to adhere to the regime and if there had been any side-effects.

You see the patient and note his blood pressure is still higher than you prefer and so decide to suggest an increase in the dose. You are able to check his renal function (which remains normal) again prior to suggesting increasing the dose by 100 per cent. The patient agrees.

c.   What is the strength of ramipril you now prescribe?
d.   How many mg of ramipril will the patient consume from this prescription until his next review in a month (28 days)?

Answers A.3

3a	1.5g
3b	21
3c	30mg
3d	42

Answers A.4

4a	14
4b	17.5mg
4c	5mg
4d	140mg

Calculation A.5

One of your patients has had a stroke and is unable to swallow tablets. The medicines on his repeat-prescribing list now need to be in liquid form. Before you write your prescription, you need to change the tablet doses to liquid doses. How many mL of each liquid will be required to provide the below doses?

Salbutamol 4mg at night

Citalopram 20mg daily

Digoxin 125 micrograms daily

Answer A.5

Salbutamol

This comes as a liquid at 2mg in 5mL, i.e., 1mg in $(5 \div 2)$mL = 1mg in 2.5mL

4mg will be in 4×2.5mL = 10mL

Citalopram

This comes as 40mg in 1mL, i.e., 1mg in $(1 \div 40)$mL = 1mg in 0.025mL

20mg will be in 20×0.025mL = 0.5mL

Digoxin

This comes as 50 micrograms in 1mL, i.e., 1 microgram in $(1 \div 50)$mL = 1 microgram in 0.02mL

125 micrograms will be in 125×0.02mL = 2.5mL

You can now write you prescription with confidence.

Numbers needed to treat NNTs

In Chapter 4, we considered different approaches to communicating risk, benefit and uncertainty. In particular, we looked at numerical depictions where numbers needed to treat were mentioned. This short section shows how to measure the NNTs.

The NNT is the number of patients you need to treat to prevent one negative outcome such as a migraine headache or diarrhoea using a particular medicine. You need a control group where the patients are not taking the medicine and a treatment group where they are. For example, if a drug has an NNT of 4 it means you have to treat four people with that drug in order to prevent the negative outcome. All you need to calculate the NNT is the absolute risk reduction (ARR); this is simply the difference between the numbers having the migraine or diarrhoea in the control group and the treatment group. Once you have this number, the NNT is the reciprocal or inverse the ARR.

So, if the number having the migraine in the control group as a percentage, to ensure the numbers in each group are equivalent, is 60 per cent (expressed as 0.6) and the number in the treatment groups is 10 per cent (expressed as 0.1), then the ARR is the reciprocal of 0.6–0.1 or 0.5 or 1/0.5 which is 2. You would need to treat only two people in order to prevent a negative outcome of, say, a migraine headache. So small numbers make you think this is an excellent drug.

Question A.1

When might this not be the case and when might a higher number be acceptable?

Answer A.1

If the drug was very effective against migraine headaches but caused other unacceptable side-effects the small number may not be clinically acceptable.

Similarly, large numbers can be acceptable if there are no other treatments available or if the existing treatment caused too many side-effects and the new one did not. In cancer treatments the NNT may be high.

From time to time, you may be discussing units of alcohol with a patient. Although this does not relate directly to prescribing, the question could arise during a consultation.

1 unit of alcohol is equivalent to 10g of alcohol.

What is the safe recommendation for units of alcohol in a week?

All adults: To keep health risks to a low level, it is safest not to drink more than 14 units per week. For adults who drink as much as 14 units per week, it is best to spread this evenly over three days or more. For the calculations below we have gone back to first principles. Let us consider some alcoholic drinks and the units they hold.

Wines are often as high as 14% w/v

Calculation A.6

How many grams of alcohol are there in a bottle of 14% wine (1 bottle contains 750 mL)? How many units of alcohol are there in this bottle?

Answer A.6

14% is 14 grams in 100mL

0.14g in 1mL

105g in a bottle (750mL)

Or 10.5 units **per bottle**

A can of lager is often 5% w/v alcohol

Calculation A.7

If a can contains 500mL of lager, how many grams of alcohol are there in the can? And how many units of alcohol are there in this can?

Answer A.7

5% is 5g in 100mL

Or 25g in a 500mL can

25g is 2.5 units per can

Spirits can be 40% v/v. A double is 50 mL

Calculation A.8

How many grams of alcohol are there in a double measure? And how many units are there in a double?

Answer A.8

100mL contains 40g of alcohol

1mL contains 40/100 or 0.4g

50mL contains 0.4 × 50 or 20g

So, each double contains two units of alcohol

Specific examples

Calculation A.9

A student drinks four pints (500mL per pint) of 4% v/v alcohol a night for a week. How many units of alcohol will he/she consume in that time?

Answer A.9

4% is:

100mL containing 4g of alcohol

1ml contains 0.04g of alcohol

The student drinks 2000mL (4 × 500mL) per night for seven nights or 14000mL

14000mL × 0.04g is 560g of alcohol

1 unit = 10g of alcohol

The student, therefore, drinks 56 units or four times the recommended amount

Calculation A.10

A lecturer drinks a bottle (750mL) of 12.5% v/v wine seven nights a week.

How many units will be consumed in a week?

Answer A.10

100ml contains 12.5mg of alcohol

1mL contains 0.125mg of alcohol

(750 × 7) 5250mL contains 5250x 0.125g or 656.25g of alcohol

The lecturer drinks 66 units a week or almost five times the recommended amount

References

Bradbury, H. and Strickland-Hodge, B. 2014. *Practical Prescribing for Medical Students.* London: Sage.

RPS 2021. *A Competency Framework for All Prescribers.* Available at www.rpharms.com/resources/frameworks/prescribing-competency-framework/competency-framework (accessed 12 May 2023).

Index

Note: Page numbers followed by "*f*" indicate figure and "*t*" indicates table.